OPHTHALMOLOGY STUDY GUIDE

For Students and Practitioners of Medicine

Fifth Edition

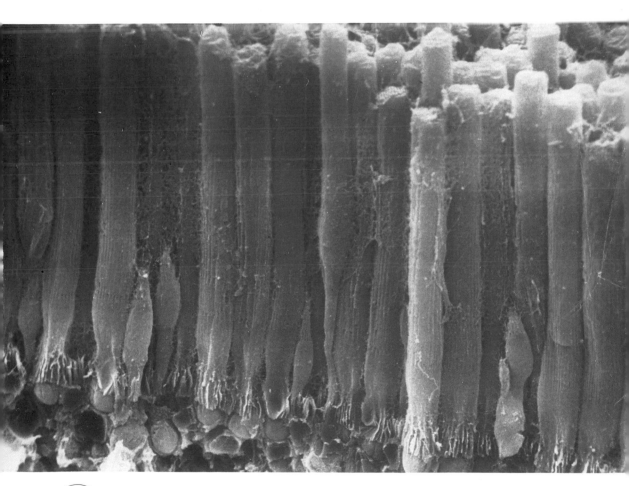

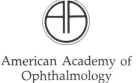

American Academy of
Ophthalmology

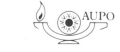

Association of University
Professors of Ophthalmology

ACKNOWLEDGMENTS: *Cover/Publication design:* Sandra Popovich, San Francisco, Yonie Overton, AAO. *Cover micrograph:* Modified with permission from Steinberg RH: Scanning electron microscopy of the bullfrog's retina and pigment epithelium. *Z. Zellforsch* 143:451-463, 1973, fig. 1. *Illustrations 1.1-1.3, 1.6; 6.1-6.3; 7.1-7.3:* Christine Gralapp, San Francisco. *Table 1.3:* Adapted with permission from Bankes JLK: *Clinical Ophthalmology.* Edinburgh, Churchill Livingstone, 1982. *Illustration 1.4:* Reprinted with permission from Appleton-Century-Crofts from Vaughan D, Asbury T: *General Ophthalmology,* ed 11. Los Altos, Calif, Lange Medical Publications, 1986. *Photograph 3.1:* Reprinted with permission from Duane TD, Jaeger EA (eds): *Clinical Ophthalmology.* Philadelphia, Harper & Row, 1985, vol 2. *Illustration 3.1:* RH Sennhenn, Burlington, Vt. *Figures 6, 7, 9, 10:* Courtesy Harry Kachadoorian. Selected figures have been reprinted from the previous edition of *Ophthalmology Study Guide,* a number of which were used with permission from The Upjohn Company and the National Medical Audiovisual Center.

Library of Congress Cataloging in Publication Data

Ophthalmology study guide for students and practitioners
    of medicine.

    Includes bibliographical references.
    1. Ophthalmology—Outlines, syllabi, etc.   I. American
Academy of Ophthalmology.   II. Association of University
Professors of Ophthalmology (U.S.).   III. Title:
Ophthalmology study guide.
RE50.064   1990   617.7   90-177
ISBN 1-56055-003-1

Fifth Edition
    First printing: 1987
    Second printing: 1990

AMERICAN ACADEMY OF OPHTHALMOLOGY

655 Beach Street
P.O. Box 7424
San Francisco, CA 94120-7424

**Ophthalmology Study Guide
was developed by the
Joint Committee on Medical Student Education
of the
American Academy of Ophthalmology
and the
Association of University Professors of Ophthalmology**

**Frank G. Berson, M.D.
Boston, MA
Executive Editor, Fifth Edition**

Henry J.L. Van Dyk, M.D., *Co-chairman*
New Orleans, LA

David E. Eifrig, M.D., *Co-chairman*
Chapel Hill, NC

Phil A. Aitken, M.D.
Burlington, VT

Edward A. Jaeger, M.D.
Philadelphia, PA

Frank G. Berson, M.D.
Boston, MA

Martha Luckenbach, M.D.
Dallas, TX

Richard D. Cunningham, M.D.
Temple, TX

Paul E. Michelson, M.D., F.A.C.S.
La Jolla, CA

John W. Gittinger, Jr., M.D.
Worcester, MA

Gary Arsham, M.D., *Consultant*
San Francisco, CA

Immediate Past Members

Guy H. Chan, M.D.; Robert S. Hepler, M.D.; Barry N. Hyman, M.D.;
Irwin E. Kanarek, M.D.; Paul R. Lichter, M.D.; David Miller, M.D.;
Charles D. Phelps, M.D.; David A. Rosen, M.D.; Melvin L. Rubin, M.D.;
Morton E. Smith, M.D.; Bruce E. Spivey, M.D.

Additional Review by

William P. Boger III, M.D.
Concord, MA

Bradford J. Shingleton, M.D.
Boston, MA

Ann Stromberg, C.O.
Boston, MA

Karla J. Johns, M.D.
Nashville, TN

Academy Staff

Suzanne K. Quick, Ph.D.
Director of Education

Yonie Overton
Project Manager

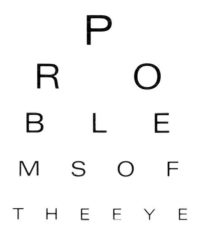

PROBLEMS OF THE EYE

Most of the things you need to know about ophthalmology, including its spelling.

OPHTHALMOLOGY STUDY GUIDE

For Students and Practitioners of Medicine

Fifth Edition

PREFACE

This study guide is designed to help you learn the most important concepts of diagnosis and management in the field of eye care. The first edition of the study guide was published in 1975. The outline presented was based on the results of the studies referenced below. In order to find out what medical students ought to know about this subject, seven common problem areas of the eye were identified and study objectives were developed for each. Through a structured response sheet,[1] these objectives were broadly distributed. Over 1,800 responses produced a surprising consensus.[2] Two further studies yielded confirmatory results.[3,4] The expanded results served as the basis for the original *Ophthalmology Study Guide*. User comments[5] have helped to update each subsequent edition.

The fifth edition employs an expanded text and a streamlined reference format. It is organized around nine chapters, each of which addresses patient problem areas with which practitioners are frequently confronted. Each chapter concludes with an annotated list of references relevant to the subject material.

Chapter One describes the general anatomy of the eye and details the steps in a basic eye examination. You will find repeated cross-references to the fundamentals established in this opening chapter. Chapters Two and Three cover acute and chronic visual loss. Chapter Two takes the form of a survey of the major disorders that can result in a sudden loss of vision. Chapter Three focuses on glaucoma, cataract, and macular degeneration.

Chapter Four discusses the red eye and how to differentiate between a minor inflammation and serious disease. Chapter Five covers ocular injuries and what to do in an emergency. The important facts about amblyopia and strabismus are summarized in Chapter Six. Chapters Seven and Eight consider ophthalmic problems as they relate to neurology and systemic disease, with Chapter Eight focusing on diabetic retinopathy. Chapter Nine covers the major ocular and systemic complications of eye drops as well as ocular complications of systemic medications.

Visuals are used throughout the current edition. Color figures depict normal and abnormal eye conditions and are also available as a companion set of seventy-five 35-mm color slides. In addition, numerous illustrations and photographs in black/white and color are used to enhance the text. Where appropriate, information is organized in tabular form to facilitate study.

Obviously, the manner in which the guide will be used will vary from school to school. Much will depend on curriculum design, on the time allocated to the subject, and on the energies of both student and teacher. Thus, the guide is intended to be a flexible instrument that summarizes the important concepts, techniques, and facts of ophthalmology for all physicians, especially those in primary care. This study guide is the product of the Joint Committee on Medical Student Education of the American Academy of Ophthalmology and the Association of University Professors of Ophthalmology. The committee anticipates that medical students will use this study guide in conjunction with the comprehensive texts and other related references annotated at the end of each chapter.

Comments on content, format, and use of this study guide are welcome. Please send them to Chairperson, Medical Student Education Committee, American Academy of Ophthalmology, P.O. Box 7424, San Francisco, California 94120-7424.

Original Research

1. Spivey BE: A technique to determine curriculum content. *J Med Ed* **46:**269–274, 1971.

2. Spivey BE: Ophthalmology for medical students: Content and comment. *Arch Ophthalmol* **84:**368–375, 1970.

3. Colenbrander A: International expectations for medical student performance in ophthalmology. *Proc Res Med Ed,* 10th Annual Conference, 1971 (AAMC).

4. Worthen DM: Ophthalmology for medical students: Objectives. *Arch Ophthalmol* **88:**314–315, 1972.

5. Waring GO III, Harris R, Walters RF, et al: Clinical ophthalmology instruction for medical students. *Surv Ophthalmol* **22:**106–112, 1977.

6. Kalina RE, Van Dyk HJL, Weinstein GW: Ophthalmology teaching in medical schools. *J Med Educ* **56:**143–145, 1981.

TEST YOUR KNOWLEDGE

Test your own initial awareness about eye care with the following 90-second quiz. It contains many statements that you have heard before.

1. Reading for prolonged periods in dim light can be harmful to the eyes.   T   F

2. Children should be taught not to hold their books too close when reading since this can harm their eyes.   T   F

3. Wearing glasses that are too strong can cause damage to the eyes.   T   F

4. If children sit too close to the television they may damage their eyes.   T   F

5. Older people who may be having trouble seeing should not use their eyes too much since they can wear them out sooner.   T   F

6. People with weak eyes should rest their eyes often in order to strengthen them.   T   F

7. Children with crossed eyes will likely outgrow this if given a little time and patience.   T   F

8. Contact lenses are good for correcting nearsightedness so that eventually neither lenses nor glasses will be needed.   T   F

9. Children who have a problem learning to read are likely to have an eye coordination problem and can be helped with special exercises.   T   F

10. Cataracts can sometimes grow back after cataract surgery.   T   F

11. Cataracts have to be "ripe" before surgery can be done.   T   F

12. Nearsighted people may outgrow their need for glasses, since they will become farsighted as they get older.   T   F

13. In older people, a sign of healthy eyes is the ability to read the newspaper without glasses.   T   F

14. People who wear glasses should be checked every year to see if a change is needed.   T   F

15. Watching a bright television picture in a dimly lighted room can be harmful to the eyes if done for long periods.   T   F

16. Ideally, more people should use an eyewash regularly to clean their eyes.   T   F

17. A blue eye should not be selected for transplantation in a brown-eyed person.   T   F

18. In rare instances, contact lenses can get lost behind the eye and even get into the brain.   T   F

19. A cataract is actually a film over the eye which can be peeled off with surgery.   T   F

20. Headaches are usually due to eyestrain.   T   F

(Answers start on page xii.)

WHO'S WHO
IN EYE CARE

The Ophthalmologist

An ophthalmologist is a physician (doctor of medicine or doctor of osteopathy) who specializes in the comprehensive care of the eyes and visual system. The ophthalmologist is the only practitioner medically trained and qualified to diagnose and treat all eye and visual system problems. Each is licensed by a state to practice medicine and surgery. Thus, an ophthalmologist is the only provider who can deliver total eye care (i.e., "vision services," contact lenses, medical eye care, and surgical eye care) as well as diagnose general diseases of the body. The ophthalmologist has completed four years of college premedical training, four years or more of medical school, one year of internship, and three or more years of specialized medical training and clinical experience in eye care.

The Optometrist

An optometrist is a health service provider who is involved with vision problems. Optometrists have not attended medical school, but they are specifically educated, trained, and state licensed to examine the eyes and to determine the presence of vision problems. Optometrists determine visual acuity and prescribe spectacles, contact lenses, and exercises. Optometrists are qualified to perform all services listed below under opticians.

The Optician

An optician is a technician who makes, verifies, and delivers to the intended wearer lenses, frames, and other specially fabricated optical devices and/or contact lenses upon prescription. The optician's functions include: prescription analysis and interpretation; determination of the lens forms best suited to the wearer's needs; the preparation and delivery of work orders for the grinding of lenses and the fabrication of eye wear; the verification of the finished ophthalmic products; the adjustment, replacement, repair, and reproduction of previously prepared ophthalmic lenses, frames, and other specially fabricated ophthalmic devices.

HOW TRUE

1. *False.* A common misconception is that the way light enters the eye is important. Except in extreme circumstances, this is just not so. Reading in dim light can no more harm the eyes than taking a photograph in dim light can harm the camera.

2. *False.* Holding books close to the eyes to read is common in children. Their eyes can accommodate (focus on near objects) easily and can keep near objects in sharp focus. No harm can come of it. In rare cases, holding a book close could be a sign of severe nearsightedness, which should be checked into; however, the habit of close reading itself will not cause nearsightedness.

3. *False.* Since glasses are something hung in front of the eyes from the nose and ears, looking through them cannot cause *harm*. A good thing to remember is that glasses treat light, not the eye. However, incorrect glasses may result in blurring, which causes discomfort and may lead to a headache.

4. *False.* Again, it is common for normal-sighted children to want to get close to the television set just as they want to get close to reading material. All individuals will hold reading material or watch television at a distance which is comfortable to them. No harm to the eyes will result.

5. *False.* The eyes are made for seeing. There is no evidence that using them for this purpose can wear them out.

6. *False.* Conversely, eyes which are "weak" for whatever reason did not get this way from overuse and can in no way be improved by rest.

7. *False.* Crossed eyes in children should *always* be considered serious; in fact, the condition *requires* referral to an ophthalmologist. Some children have *apparent* but not truly crossed eyes. In such cases, the apparent crossing is due to a broad bridge to the nose. As the nose matures, this apparent crossing will lessen and disappear. However, truly crossed eyes should never be ignored in the hope that the crossing will disappear with time.

8. *False.* Only *incorrectly* fitted contact lenses can change the shape of the cornea to give the appearance of having corrected myopia. Intentionally fitting contact lenses in an incorrect manner is considered risky since permanent harm to the eyes has been known to result from improperly fitted lenses.

9. *False.* The misconception that reading problems are due to poor eye coordination is perpetrated either intentionally or naively by some educators and nonmedical practitioners. All controlled studies have proved this statement to be blatantly false. Unfortunately, believing or desperate parents provide great economic incentive to those who treat on this premise.

10. *False.* Since a cataract is an opacity in the lens of the eye, the cataract cannot grow back when the entire lens is removed (intracapsular extraction). However, the posterior capsule of the lens may opacify when the lens is not completely removed (extracapsular extraction).

11. *False.* Lenses are not like fruit on the vine. The indication for cataract surgery rests largely on the visual impairment caused by the cataract and not on any criteria used for the harvest.

12. *False.* *All* individuals become presbyopic with age. This has nothing to do with nearsightedness or farsightedness.

13. *False.* Individuals who are nearsighted to a certain extent can always read without glasses no matter what their age. Sometimes a cataract will cause an eye to become nearsighted, giving what has been referred to as "second sight." Thus, the ability to read without glasses in old age indicates nearsightedness, either present since youth or due to cataract.

14. *False.* Glasses have nothing to do with the health of the eyes. As long as an individual is happy with his vision with the present glasses, there is little reason to check for change. This is somewhat analogous to going to the shoe store each year to see if you need a new pair of shoes.

15. *False.* Just as in some earlier questions, the misconception is that the eye will be *harmed* by the way light enters it. The eye merely deals with light regardless of contrast. If an individual does not like the marked contrast of a bright television picture in a dimly lighted room, the individual can turn on some lights. It is important to distinguish between harm and *discomfort*.

16. *False.* The only thing to be said about eyewash is the less put into the eyes, the better.

17. *False.* Only corneas can be transplanted, and the cornea is colorless in all eyes.

18. *False.* The conjunctiva prevents a contact lens from passing behind the eye.

19. *False.* A common misconception is that a cataract is a "growth" or "film" which covers the eye. A cataract is merely an imperfection in the transparency of the normal lens of the eye. If the transparency is impaired to the point of significant visual impairment, the entire lens is removed from the eye. Nothing is "peeled" away.

20. *False.* Headaches usually do not occur on an ocular basis.

You will be able to find greater rationale for these answers in the various chapters of the study guide and in the references cited at the end of each chapter.

CONTENTS

FIGURE LIST

The Tables

The Photos

The Illustrations

The Figures
(Note: Numbers correspond to both text and slide set.)

- Lens: transparent, biconvex body located behind the pupil and iris, part of the refracting mechanism of the eye.
- Ciliary body: produces aqueous humor and suspends the lens via tiny ligaments called zonules. Contraction of the ciliary muscle permits focusing of the lens.
- Posterior chamber: the small space behind the iris and in front of the zonules where the aqueous humor is produced.
- Vitreous cavity: the large space (4.5 cc) behind the lens that extends up to the retina. The cavity is filled with a transparent jelly-like material called vitreous humor.
- Retina: the neural tissue lining the vitreous cavity posteriorly. Essentially transparent except for the blood vessels on its inner surface, the retina sends the initial visual signal to the brain via the optic nerve.
- Macula: the area of the retina in the posterior pole responsible for fine, central vision. The oval depression in the center of the macula is called the fovea.
- Choroid: the vascular, pigmented tissue layer between the sclera and retina. The choroid provides the blood supply for the outer retinal layers.
- Optic disc: the portion of the optic nerve visible within the eye. It is comprised of axons whose cell bodies are located in the ganglion cell layer of the retina.

Optics

The cornea and the lens make up the refractive surface of the eye. The cornea refracts approximately two thirds of the light entering the eye and the lens approximately one third to form an image on the retina. Reduced visual acuity will result if the axial length of the eye is either too short (i.e., hyperopia; also called hypermetropia) or too long (i.e., myopia) for the refracting power of the cornea and lens. Visual acuity is also reduced if the refracting power of the cornea and lens is different in one meridian than in another (i.e., astigmatism). These optical defects can be corrected by the use of either spectacle lenses or contact lenses. A pinhole placed directly in front of the eye will narrow the pupillary aperture and thereby minimize the blurring induced by a refractive error.

The ability of the ciliary muscle to contract and the lens to become more convex is called accommodation. With increasing age, the lens of every eye suffers a progressive hardening with loss of ability to change its shape. Loss of accommodation is manifested by a decreased ability to focus on near objects (i.e., presbyopia), while corrected distance visual acuity remains normal. Presbyopia develops progressively with age but becomes clinically manifest in the early to midforties, when the ability to accommodate at reading distance (thirty-five to forty centimeters) is lost. Presbyopia is corrected by spectacle lenses, either as reading glasses or as the lower segment of bifocal lenses, the upper segment of which can contain a correction for distance visual acuity if needed. Some presbyopic myopes will simply remove their distance glasses to read, since they will not need to accommodate in an uncorrected state.

Visual Acuity Defined

Visual acuity is a measurement of the smallest object a person can identify at a given distance from the eye.

Common Abbreviations. The following are common abbreviations used to discuss visual acuity:

    VA: visual acuity
    OD *(oculus dexter)*: right eye
    OS *(oculus sinister)*: left eye
    OU *(oculus uterque)*: both eyes

Color Vision

The normal retina contains three color-sensitive pigments: red sensitive, green sensitive, and blue sensitive. A developmental deficiency in either concentration or function of one or more of these pigments causes various combinations and degrees of congenital color vision defects. Most such defects occur in males through an X-linked inheritance pattern. Color vision abnormalities also may be acquired in individuals with retinal or optic nerve disorders *(see Chapter 7, Neuro-Ophthalmology).*

Intraocular Pressure

Intraocular pressure (IOP) is determined largely by the outflow of aqueous humor from the eye. The greater the resistance to outflow, the higher the intraocular pressure. Alterations in the actual production of aqueous humor will have an effect on the intraocular pressure.

Intraocular pressure varies among individuals. An IOP of 15 mm Hg represents the mean IOP in a "normal" population. However, an IOP in the range of 10 to 21.5 mm Hg is acceptable, and falls within two standard deviations of the mean.

When to Examine

All patients should have an eye examination as part of a physical examination by the primary care physician. Essential equipment for an eye examination consists of a few items which can be transported, if necessary, with other medical instruments **(Photo 1.1).** Visual acuity, pupillary reactions, extraocular movements, and direct ophthalmoscopy through an undilated pupil comprise a minimal examination. Distance visual acuity measurement

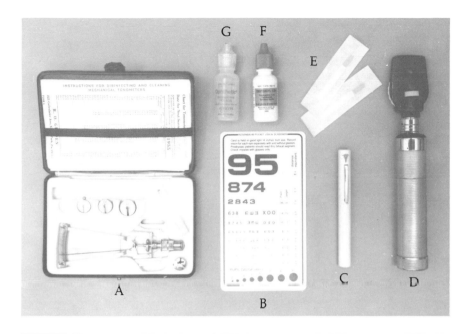

Photo 1.1. Essential equipment for basic eye examination. Includes a Schiotz tonometer (A), near vision card (B), penlight (C), direct ophthalmoscope (D), fluorescein strips (E), mydriatic (F), and topical anesthetic (G).

should be performed in all children as soon as possible after the third birthday because of the importance of early detection of amblyopia. The single E chart *(see Chapter 6, Amblyopia and Strabismus)* is used in place of the standard Snellen eye chart.

Under certain conditions, additional tests may be indicated. (Details on how to perform these and other tests can be found in the sections, *How to Examine* and *Other Examination Techniques.)*

- Schiotz tonometry should be performed on patients over the age of forty since the incidence of glaucoma increases with age, or on any patient for whom the diagnosis of glaucoma is suspected.

- Fluorescein staining of the cornea is necessary to look for a suspected epithelial defect or abnormality.

- Eversion of the upper lid is necessary to search for a suspected foreign body.

- Pupillary dilation is required in cases of unexplained visual loss or when fundus pathology is suspected (e.g., diabetes mellitus).

- Color vision testing may be part of an eye examination when requested by the patient or by another agency, and in patients with retinal or optic nerve disorders.

- Confrontation visual field testing to look for a suspected field defect may be suggested by the patient's history and/or symptoms.

How to Examine

Distance Visual Acuity

Distance visual acuity is recorded as a ratio or fraction comparing patient performance to an agreed upon standard. In this notation, the first number represents the distance separating the patient and the eye chart (usually the Snellen eye chart, **Photo 1.2**); the second number represents the distance at which the letters being read can be seen by a person with normal acuity. Visual acuity of 20/80 thus indicates that the patient can recognize at twenty feet a symbol that can be recognized by a person with normal acuity at eighty feet.

Visual acuity of 20/20 represents normal visual acuity. Many "normal" individuals actually see better than 20/20, for example, at 20/15 or even 20/12. If this is the case, one should record it as such.

Alternative notations are the internationally preferred decimal notation (e.g., 20/20 = 1.0, 20/40 = 0.5, 20/200 = 0.1) and notation in meters (e.g., 20/20 = 6/6, 20/100 = 6/30).

Visual acuity is tested most often at a distance of twenty feet, or six meters. Greater distances are cumbersome and impractical; and, at shorter distances, variations in the test distance assume greater proportional significance. For practical purposes, a distance of six meters may be equated with optical infinity.

Conventional Snellen Eye Chart

- *Step 1.* Place the patient at the designated distance, usually twenty feet or six meters, from a well-illuminated Snellen chart (**see Photo 1.2**). The patient should wear his glasses if they are normally worn for distance vision.

- *Step 2.* Completely occlude the left eye using an opaque occluder or the palm of your hand, or by having the patient cover his own eye.

- *Step 3.* Ask the patient to read the smallest line in which he can distinguish more than one half of the letters. If the single E chart is being used, have the patient designate the direction in which the strokes of the E point.

- *Step 4.* Record the acuity measurement as a notation (e.g., 20/20) in which the first number represents the distance at which the test is performed and the second number represents the numerical designation for the line read.

- *Step 5.* Repeat the procedure for the fellow eye. By convention, the right eye is tested and recorded first.

- *Step 6.* If visual acuity is 20/40 or less in one or both eyes, repeat the test, but with the subject viewing the test chart through a pinhole occluder, and record these results. The pinhole occluder may be used over the subject's glasses.

If a patient cannot see the largest Snellen letters, proceed as follows.

- *Step 1.* Reduce the distance between patient and chart. Record the new distance as the numerator of the acuity designation (e.g., 5/70, equivalent to 20/280).

- *Step 2.* If the patient is unable to see the largest Snellen letter at three feet, ask him to count the fingers held up on one of your hands. Record the distance at which counting is done accurately: CF 10 ft.

- *Step 3.* If the patient cannot count fingers, determine whether or not he can detect the movement of your hand. Record a positive response as hand motion: HM 5 ft.

- *Step 4.* If the patient cannot detect hand motion, use a penlight to determine whether he can detect the presence or direction of light. Record the patient's response as LP (light perception), LP with projection (able to distinguish the direction of the light), or NLP (no light perception).

The term visual acuity impairment (or simply visual impairment) is used to describe a condition of the eyes. Visual disability describes a condition of the individual. The disabling effect of an impairment depends in part on the individual's ability to adapt and to compensate. Two individuals with the same visual impairment measured on a Snellen eye chart may show very different levels of visual disability. **Table 1.1** summarizes the differences between visual acuity impairment and visual disability.

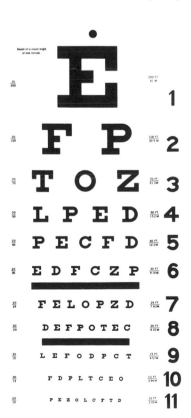

Photo 1.2. Snellen eye chart

Table 1.1. Visual Acuity Impairment Versus Visual Disability

Visual Acuity Impairment	Visual Disability	Comment
20/12 to 20/25	Normal vision	Healthy young adults average better than 20/20 acuity
20/30 to 20/70	Near-normal	Causes no serious problems, but vision should be explored for potential improvement or possible early disease. Most states will issue a driver's license to individuals with this level of vision in at least one eye.
20/80 to 20/160	Moderate low vision	Strong reading glasses or magnifiers usually provide adequate reading speed. But usually insufficient for a driver's license.
20/200 to 20/400 or CF 10 ft.	Severe low vision; legally blind by U.S. definition	Gross orientation and mobility generally adequate, but difficulty with traffic signs, bus numbers, etc. Reading requires high power magnifiers. Reading speed and endurance reduced.
CF 8 ft. to 4 ft.	Profound low vision	Increasing problems with visual orientation and mobility. Long cane useful to explore environment. Highly motivated and persistent individuals can read visually with extreme magnification. Others rely on nonvisual means: braille, "talking books," radio.
less than CF 4 ft.	Near blindness	Vision unreliable, except under ideal circumstances. Must rely on nonvisual aids.
NLP	Total blindness	No light perception. Must rely entirely on other senses.

Near Visual Acuity

Near visual acuity testing may be performed if the patient has a complaint about near vision. Otherwise, testing "at near" is performed only if distance testing is difficult or impossible—at the patient's bedside, for instance. In such situations, testing with a near card may be the only feasible way to determine visual acuity.

Testing. If a patient normally wears glasses for reading, he should wear them during testing. This holds true for presbyopic patients in particular. The patient holds the test card, for example, a Rosenbaum Pocket Vision Screener **(Photo 1.3),** at the distance specified on the card. This distance is usually fourteen inches or thirty-five centimeters. While the examiner occludes one of the patient's eyes, the patient reads the smallest characters legible on the card. The test is then repeated for the fellow eye.

Recording. Letter size designations and test distances vary. To avoid ambiguity, both should be recorded: J5 at 14 in, 6 point at 40 cm. Some near cards carry *distance equivalent* values. These are only valid if the test is done at the recommended distance. If a standard near vision card is not available, any printed matter such as a telephone book or newspaper may be substituted. Both the approximate type size read and the distance at which the material was held are recorded.

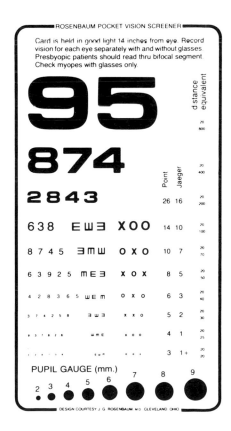

Photo 1.3.
Rosenbaum pocket vision screener

Estimating Visual Acuity in the Uncooperative Patient

(See Chapter 6, Amblyopia and Strabismus, for the testing of infants and toddlers.)

Withdrawal or a change in facial expression in response to light or sudden movement indicates the presence of vision. A brisk pupillary response to light also suggests the presence of vision. The exception to this is the patient with cortical blindness, which is due to bilateral widespread destruction of the visual cortex. If there is any doubt, referral to an ophthalmologist is recommended.

Confrontation Fields

The examiner takes a position in front of the patient. The patient is asked to cover the left eye with the palm of the left hand; the examiner closes his right eye. Thus, the field of the examiner's left eye is used as a reference in assessing the field of the patient's right eye. The patient is asked to "count the fingers" of the examiner in each of the four quadrants of the visual field. Wiggling the fingers as a visual stimulus is not desirable. After the patient's right eye is tested, the procedure is repeated for the left eye with the patient covering the right eye with the palm of the right hand, and the examiner closing his left eye.

Color Vision Testing

Color vision testing is performed with the use of pseudoisochromatic plates (e.g., Ishihara plates) that present numbers or figures against a background of colored dots. The person with abnormal color discrimination will be confused by the pseudoisochromatic plates, which force a choice based on hue discrimination alone while concealing other clues such as brightness, saturation, and contours.

The patient should wear glasses during testing if they are normally worn for near vision. The agency for which the test is done ordinarily will request that both eyes be tested together, but, on occasion, may request that each eye be tested separately.

The color plates are presented consecutively under good illumination, preferably natural light. Results are recorded according to the detailed instructions provided with the plates. Usually, a fraction is specified, with the numerator equivalent to the number of correct responses and the denominator the total plates presented. The type of color defect can be determined by recording the specific errors and using the instructions provided with the plates.

Amsler Grid Testing

Amsler grid testing is a method of evaluating the macula. *(See Chapter 3, Chronic Visual Loss, for details and a visual, Photo 3.3.)*

Measurement of Intraocular Pressure

There are a number of instruments for measuring intraocular pressure. The Schiotz tonometer **(see Photo 1.1)** is the instrument of choice for the

Table 1.2. Calibration Scale for Schiotz Tonometers

	Plunger Load (gms)			
	5.5	7.5	10.0	15.0
Scale Reading (scale units)	Intraocular Pressure (mm Hg)			
0	41	59	82	127
0.5	38	51	75	118
1.0	35	50	70	109
1 5	32	46	64	101
2.0	29	42	59	94
2.5	27	39	55	88
3.0	24	36	51	82
3.5	22	33	47	76
4.0	21	30	43	71
4.5	19	28	40	66
5.0	17	26	37	62
5.5	16	24	34	58
6.0	15	??	32	54
6 5	13	20	29	50
7.0	12	19	27	46
7.5	11	17	25	43
8.0	10	16	23	40
8.5	9	14	21	38
9.0	9	13	20	35
9.5	8	12	18	32
10.0	7	11	16	30
10.5	6	10	15	27
11.0	6	9	14	25
11.5	5	8	13	23
12.0		8	11	21
12.5		7	10	20
13.0		6	10	18
13.5		6	9	17
14.0		5	8	15
14.5			7	14
15.0			6	13
15.5			6	11
16.0			5	10
16.5				9
17.0				8
17.5				8
18.0				7

primary care physician. It is readily available at low cost, and the technique is easy to perform on most adult patients in either an outpatient setting or at the bedside. When a tonometer with a given weight is placed on the anesthetized cornea, the cornea is indented in an amount related to the intraocular pressure. The Schiotz tonometer has a scale that indicates the degree of actual indentation. When the amount of weight is known and the Schiotz tonometer is used to measure the indentation, the intraocular pressure can be read from the printed conversion table **(Table 1.2)** that comes with the tonometer. The less indentation, the lower the scale reading and the higher the intraocular pressure.

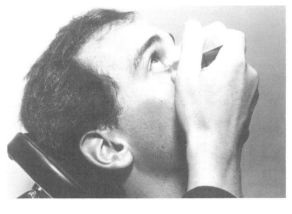

A

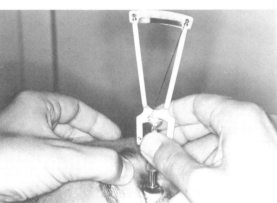

B

Photo 1.4. Technique for Schiotz tonometry. (A) Topical anesthetic is instilled. (B) Lids are separated and tonometer positioned just above the eye. (C) Tonometer is lowered onto the cornea and the scale reading noted. (D) Procedure is repeated for the fellow eye.

Schiotz Tonometry

- *Step 1.* Ask the patient to assume a supine position, and anesthetize the cornea with topical proparacaine hydrochloride 0.5% (*Ophthaine®*) or an equivalent **(Photo 1.4A).**

- *Step 2.* The tonometer is used initially with the 5.5 gram weight in place.

- *Step 3.* Have the patient fixate on a spot above his line of vision, or on the thumb of his upheld hand. Gently spread the lids of the right eye against the bony margin of the orbit; do not apply pressure to the globe itself. Hold the tonometer as perpendicular as possible just above the eye until the patient seems relaxed **(Photo 1.4B).**

- *Step 4.* Gently lower the tonometer onto the cornea for a few seconds to determine the scale reading **(Photo 1.4C).**

- *Step 5.* Repeat the procedure in the fellow eye **(Photo 1.4D).**

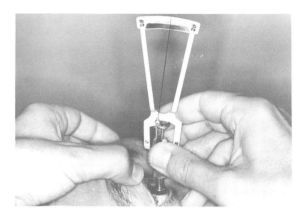

C

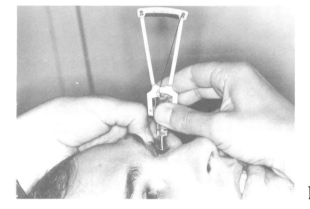

D

- *Step 6.* If the scale reading is 3 units or less for either eye, repeat the measurement. Add weights to the 5.5 gram weight—to a total of 7.5, 10.0, or 15.0 grams as necessary—to reach a scale reading in the range of 3.5 to 8.0 units. The repetition is done to double check one's findings, since a scale reading of 3.0 units or less indicates an elevated IOP.

- *Step 7.* Refer to the calibration scale for Schiotz tonometers **(see Table 1.2)** to determine the intraocular pressure for a scale reading at a particular plunger load.

  For example, at a plunger load of 5.5 grams, a scale reading of 4.5 units would indicate an intraocular pressure of 19 mm Hg, which is within the normal range of 10.0 to 21.5 mm Hg. As the table shows, a scale reading of 3.0 units or less with a 5.5 gram weight indicates an elevated intraocular pressure.

- *Step 8.* Carefully clean the tonometer after each use to prevent office transmission of disease, such as viral conjunctivitis, to other patients. To clean, first disassemble the tonometer. Clean the barrel first with a pipe cleaner soaked in alcohol, then with a dry pipe cleaner. Clean the footplate with an alcohol swab. All tonometer surfaces must be allowed to dry before reassembling. Disposable tonometer covers are also available.

Precautions. Topical anesthetic drops have little effect on the margins of the eyelids. Thus, if the tonometer touches the lids, the patient will feel it and squeeze. Such an occurrence must be avoided by holding the lids widely apart.

There is hardly any circumstance in tonometry screening where a falsely low reading occurs. Holding the eyelids apart improperly would result in a falsely high reading only if digital pressure were applied on the eyeball through the lids.

Although it is not uncommon to roughen the corneal epithelium during Schiotz tonometry, only careless technique or preexisting corneal disease could result in significant damage to the epithelium; such occurrences are unusual.

Assessing Anterior Chamber Depth

Principle. When the anterior chamber is shallow, the iris becomes convex as it is bowed forward over the lens. Under these conditions, the nasal iris is seen in shadow when a light is directed from the opposite side **(Illus. 1.4).** As the shallowness of the anterior chamber increases, so do the convexity of the iris and the shaded view of the nasal iris. A shallow anterior chamber may indicate narrow-angle glaucoma (also called angle-closure glaucoma) or a narrow angle that could close with pupillary dilation.

Method. Shine a light from the temporal side of the head across the front of the eye parallel to the plane of the iris. Look at the nasal aspect of the iris. If two thirds or more of the nasal iris is in shadow, the chamber is probably shallow and the angle narrow. If you are unsure as to the extent of shadow, direct the light more from the front of the eye, since this will eliminate shadows entirely. Repeat the test for the fellow eye.

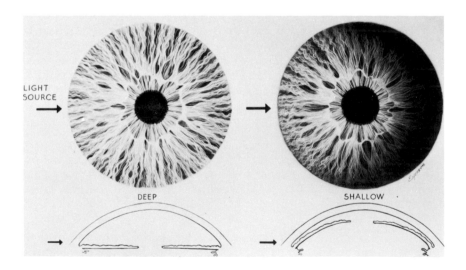

Illus. 1.4. Estimation of anterior chamber depth

Ophthalmoscopy

When examining the patient's right eye, the direct ophthalmoscope is held in the right hand and the right eye is used to view the patient's eye. The examiner uses his left hand and his left eye to examine the patient's left eye. The patient's spectacles are usually removed, and, barring astigmatic refractive errors, most examiners prefer to remove their own glasses as well. Contact lenses worn by either patient or examiner may be left in place.

Dilating the pupil. Pharmacologic dilation of the patient's pupils will greatly facilitate ophthalmoscopy. Recommended agents include either tropicamide 1% (*Mydriacyl®*) or phenylephrine hydrochloride 2.5% (*Ak-Dilate®*) (*see Chapter 9, Drugs and the Eye*). Dilation of the pupil should not be done under the following conditions.

- *Condition 1.* Do not dilate if assessment of anterior chamber depth suggests a shallow chamber and a narrow angle, because an attack of angle-closure glaucoma might be precipitated.

- *Condition 2.* If a patient is undergoing neurological observation and pupillary signs are being followed (e.g., a head-injured patient), do not dilate until the neurologist or neurosurgeon thinks it is safe to do so.

- *Condition 3.* Do not dilate if a patient has had a cataract extraction with implantation of an intraocular lens that is *iris supported* because the lens implant could dislocate. The iris-supported intraocular lens was a popular implant at one time, but is no longer used by most ophthalmic surgeons. The pupil in such a patient is usually square-shaped.

Red reflex. Light reflected off the fundus of the patient produces a red reflex when viewed through the ophthalmoscope at a distance of one foot. A normal red reflex **(Fig. 1)** is evenly colored and is not interrupted by shadows. Opacities in the media appear as black silhouettes and can be best appreciated when the pupil has been dilated (*see Chapter 3, Chronic Visual Loss, Fig. 17*). The patient's eye is approached as closely as possible and the power of the lenses in the ophthalmoscope is reduced until the optic disc comes into focus. The optic disc, retinal blood vessels, retinal background, and macula are then examined in that order.

Optic disc. In most cases, when viewed through the ophthalmoscope, the normal optic disc **(Fig. 2)** is slightly oval in the vertical meridian and has a pink color due to capillarity. There is a central depression in the surface of the disc called the physiologic cup. The optic disc can be thought of as the "yardstick" of the ocular fundus. Lesions seen with the ophthalmoscope are measured in disc diameters.

A great deal of normal variation exists in the appearance of the optic disc. The size of the physiologic cup varies among individuals. (*But see Chapter 3, Chronic Visual Loss, for a discussion of glaucomatous cupping.*) The pigmented coats of the eye—the retinal pigment epithelium and the choroid—frequently fail to reach the margin of the optic disc, producing a hypopigmented crescent **(Fig. 3).** Such crescents are especially common in myopic eyes on the temporal side of the optic disc.

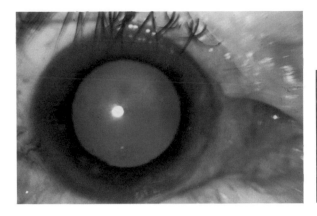

Fig. 1. Red reflex. Reddish light reflected from the fundus can be visible even at a distance of 1 or 2 feet when the direction of illumination and the direction of observation approach each other — a condition that can be achieved with the ophthalmoscope.

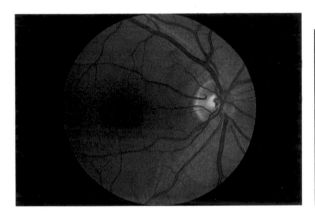

Fig. 2. Normal posterior pole. A normal optic disc is shown, with a small central physiologic cup and healthy neural rim. Major branches of the central retinal artery emanate from the disc, whereas the major branches of the central retinal vein collect at the disc. Temporal to the disc is the macula, which appears darker with no blood vessels present in the center.

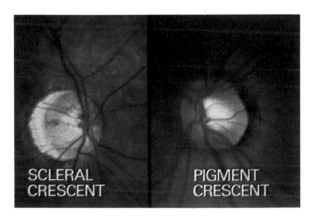

SCLERAL CRESCENT   PIGMENT CRESCENT

Fig. 3. Scleral crescent/Pigment crescent. This figure shows normal variants of the disc. On the left, retinal and choroidal pigmentation do not reach the disc margin, leaving an exposed white scleral crescent. On the right, pigment accumulation is seen at the disc margin.

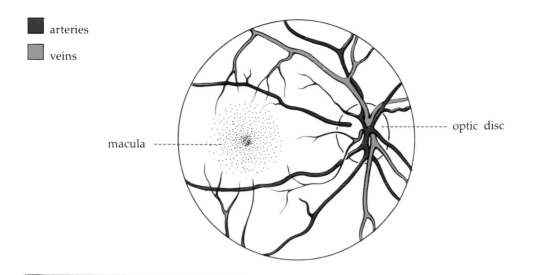

arteries

veins

macula ------------

optic disc

Illus. 1.5. Fundus diagram

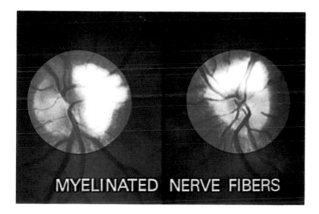

MYELINATED NERVE FIBERS

Fig. 4. Myelinated nerve fibers. Usually, the axons of the retinal ganglion cells acquire myelin sheaths only behind the optic disc. Occasionally, as a normal variant, myelin may be deposited along axons at the border of the disc or even away from the disc elsewhere in the retina. These white, feathery patterns may be mistaken for papilledema. (The illuminated circle represents the field of view of the ophthalmoscope.)

Conversely, an excess of pigment may be seen in some eyes, producing a heavily pigmented margin along the optic disc **(see Fig. 3).** The retinal nerve fibers (i.e., ganglion cell axons) ordinarily are nonmyelinated at the optic disc and retina, but occasionally myelination **(Fig. 4)** may extend on to the surface of the optic disc and retina, producing a dense, white superficial opacification.

Retinal circulation. The retinal circulation is composed of arteries and veins, visible with the ophthalmoscope **(compare Illus. 1.5 with Fig. 2).** The central retinal artery branches at or on the optic disc into divisions that supply the four quadrants of the inner retinal layers; these divisions lie superficially in the nerve fiber layer. A similarly arranged system of retinal veins collects at the optic disc where spontaneous pulsation (with collapse during systole) may be observed in eighty percent of normal eyes. The ratio of normal vein to artery diameter is 3:2. The examiner should follow arteries out from the disc and veins back to the disc in each quadrant, noting in particular arterio-venous (A-V) crossing phenomena.

Macula. The normal macula **(see Illus. 1.5 and Fig. 2),** located directly temporal to the optic disc, usually appears darker than the surrounding retina because the specialized retinal pigment epithelium cells of the macula are taller and more heavily pigmented. In some eyes the macula may appear slightly yellow. This phenomenon, known as *macula lutea,* is due to the yellow pigment xanthophyll in the retina. The central depression of the fovea may act as a concave mirror during ophthalmoscopy and produce a light reflection known as the foveal reflex.

Retinal background. The normal retinal background is a uniform red-orange color, due primarily to the pigmentation of the retinal pigment epithelium. The blood and pigment of the choroid also contribute to the appearance of the retinal background. For example, in heavily pigmented races the ocular fundus has a darker color due to increased choroidal pigment content. The *periphery* is the anterior area of the fundus not visible when the vessel and macula examinations are done with a direct ophthalmoscope.

Pupillary Testing

Inspection of the pupils should be part of the screening physical examination. Inspection should include testing the patient's direct and consensual pupillary reactions to light, with the patient looking at a distant object. Occasionally, this examination may reveal indications of neurologic disease. *(See Chapter 7, Neuro-Ophthalmology, for a description of the swinging flashlight test for the detection of an afferent defect in the anterior visual pathway.)* More frequently, pupillary inspection points up active or prior ocular disease by revealing alterations in pupillary shape or size which are the result of local intraocular effects (e.g., damage to the pupillary sphincter or adhesions of the iris to the lens).

Table 1.3. Cardinal Fields of Gaze

LOOKING RIGHT AND UP	**LOOKING LEFT AND UP**
R. superior rectus	L. superior rectus
L. inferior oblique	R. inferior oblique
LOOKING RIGHT	**LOOKING LEFT**
R. lateral rectus	L. lateral rectus
L. medial rectus	R. medial rectus
LOOKING RIGHT AND DOWN	**LOOKING LEFT AND DOWN**
R. inferior rectus	L. inferior rectus
L. superior oblique	R. superior oblique

Testing Eye Movements

The patient is asked to follow an object in six directions, the cardinal fields of gaze **(Table 1.3)**: (1) right; (2) right and up; (3) right and down; (4) left; (5) left and up; and (6) left and down. This enables the examiner to systematically test each muscle in its primary field of action and thus detect a possible isolated weakness or paralysis. *(See Chapter 6, Amblyopia and Strabismus, for a description of the cover test for the detection of strabismus, a misalignment of the two eyes.)*

Other Examination Techniques

Eversion of the Upper Lid

The patient is asked to look downward and the examiner grasps the eyelashes of the upper lid between the thumb and index finger. A cotton-tipped applicator is used to press gently downward over the superior aspect of the tarsal plate as the lid margin is pulled upward by the lashes. Pressure is maintained on the everted upper lid while the patient is encouraged to keep looking downward. The examiner should have a penlight within reach to inspect the exposed conjunctival surface of the upper lid for a foreign body or other abnormality. To return the lid to its normal position, the examiner releases the lid margin and the patient is instructed to look upward.

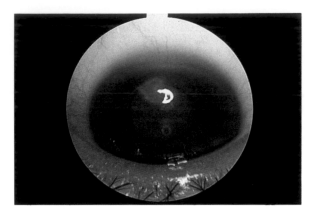

Fig. 5. Fluorescein stain. A corneal abrasion is delineated by fluorescein stain, which marks any area denuded of epithelium. Irregularity of the corneal surface is indicated by the distorted light reflection.

Fluorescein Staining of the Cornea

Fluorescein is applied in the form of a sterile filter paper strip, which is moistened with a drop of water or saline and then touched to the conjunctiva. A few blinks spread the fluorescein over the cornea. Areas of bright green staining denote absent or diseased epithelium **(Fig. 5).** Viewing the eye under cobalt blue light enhances the visibility of the fluorescence.

Two precautions to keep in mind when using fluorescein are (1) using fluorescein impregnated strips instead of stock solutions of fluorescein because such solutions are susceptible to contamination with *Pseudomonas* species; and (2) having the patient remove soft contact lenses prior to application to avoid discoloration.

Summary of the Basic Eye Examination

- *Step 1.* Measure the visual acuity for each eye.
- *Step 2.* Perform a confrontation field for each eye.
- *Step 3.* Inspect the lids and the surrounding tissues.
- *Step 4.* Test the extraocular movements.
- *Step 5.* Test the pupils for direct and consensual responses.
- *Step 6.* Inspect the conjunctiva and sclera.
- *Step 7.* Inspect the cornea.
- *Step 8.* Assess the anterior chamber for depth and clarity.

- *Step 9.* Inspect the iris.
- *Step 10.* Assess the lens for clarity through direct ophthalmoscopy.
- *Step 11.* Use the ophthalmoscope to study the fundus, including the disc, vessels, and macula.
- *Step 12.* Perform Schiotz tonometry.

Management or Referral

Reduced Visual Acuity

The guidelines discussed below apply for patients in whom reduced visual acuity (VA) is found, unless the patient has been seen by an ophthalmologist and the condition has been confirmed as stable.

VA less than 20/20. Any patient with visual acuity less than 20/20 in one or both eyes should be referred to an ophthalmologist if visual symptoms are present. Reduced visual acuity is the best single criterion by which to differentiate potentially blinding conditions from trivial ocular disorders .

VA less than 20/40. Any patient with visual acuity of 20/40 or less in both eyes is an equally important candidate for referral, even in the absence of complaints. Although many such patients will be suffering only from uncorrected refractive errors, undetected painless progressive loss of vision does occur in many disorders of the eyes and visual system.

Asymmetry. Any patient with a difference in visual acuity between the two eyes of two lines or more on the Snellen chart should be referred promptly, even if visual acuity in one or both eyes is better than 20/40. Generally, visual function is nearly identical between the two eyes; thus, in the absence of known causes of reduced vision, asymmetry of visual acuity may be a harbinger of disease.

Presbyopia. Presbyopia is manifested by reduced near vision with no change in distance visual acuity. Middle-aged or elderly patients complaining of this combination will benefit from a referral for the prescription of corrective lenses.

Appearance of the Fundus

Numerous fundus examinations will be required in order to recognize the great range of normal ophthalmoscopic appearances. When an abnormality is suspected, further studies or consultation may be required since fundus abnormalities may indicate significant ocular or systemic diseases. Ophthalmologic consultation should be sought for fundus changes accompanied by acute visual complaints.

Photographs of the ocular fundus are taken with a camera that provides a greater field of view than is possible with the direct ophthalmoscope. Many ocular fundus abnormalities have three-dimensional qualities, such as elevation or depression, but the examiner is limited to a monocular, two-dimensional ophthalmoscopic view. It is necessary to learn to think in three dimensions in order to grasp the pathophysiology.

Intraocular Pressure

A patient with a Schiotz tension of 22 mm Hg or greater (i.e., a scale reading of 3.5 units or lower, using the 5.5-gram weight) should be referred to an ophthalmologist for further evaluation.

Points to Remember

- *Point 1.* Testing the visual acuity of a patient without his glasses at a distance at which glasses normally are worn wastes the time of the patient and the examiner (unless the glasses are unavailable).

- *Point 2.* Although bifocal spectacles usually are considered reading aids, the upper segment of the bifocal lens frequently contains a correction which improves distance vision as well.

- *Point 3.* Patients may read the visual acuity chart with both eyes, either intentionally or unintentionally, if the examiner does not take care to see that one eye is completely occluded.

- *Point 4.* A patient will often read additional, smaller letters on the chart with encouragement by the examiner, thereby increasing the accuracy of the examination data.

- *Point 5.* A well-lighted hallway often provides an acceptable location for distance visual acuity testing.

- *Point 6.* Nurses are often trained to assess visual acuity as part of a general physical examination.

- *Point 7.* Visual acuity screening of preschool children is the only means of detecting remediable failure of visual development (i.e., amblyopia).

- *Point 8.* After the third birthday, children will learn the single E visual acuity test remarkably quickly, either in the physician's office or with prior instruction in the home.

- *Point 9.* When performing tonometry, it is essential to hold the lids apart by holding them firmly against the bony margin of the orbit rather than by forcing them against the globe.

- *Point 10.* If the pupils are equal and the reactions to light are brisk and equal, testing of pupillary response to accommodation (i.e., at near) will never reveal abnormalities and is not necessary.

Sample Problems

Sample Cases With Commentary

1. A fourteen-year-old boy is seen for a physical examination at school. He admits to difficulty in reading the blackboard but not in reading textbooks. He does not wear glasses.

   Examination Data:

   Visual acuity (VA): Right eye (OD) 20/100; pinhole 20/25
   Left eye (OS) 20/100; pinhole 20/25

   Comment: The combination of decreased distance vision with preserved near vision is typical of myopia, which often becomes symptomatic during adolescence. Presumptive evidence of refractive error is provided by the marked improvement in visual acuity that occurs with the use of the pinhole. Note that visual acuity with pinhole frequently does not reach 20/20. The patient should be referred to an ophthalmologist as a regular rather than an urgent consultation.

2. A seventy-eight-year-old woman is seen for an annual physical examination and complains of mild difficulty in reading and seeing street signs.

   Examination Data:

   VA (with bifocals): OD 20/50; no improvement with pinhole
   OS 20/40; no improvement with pinhole

   Ophthalmoscopy: lens opacity, each eye

   Comment: Cataract is a common cause of painless progressive loss of vision in older individuals. On further questioning, this particular patient related that six months previously she had seen an ophthalmologist who had also diagnosed cataract. Surgery was deferred because the patient believed that the visual handicap was not sufficiently severe to warrant surgery. Referral is not required since the cause of visual loss has been established and since the patient is under the care of an ophthalmologist.

3. A forty-year-old man is seen for an annual executive physical. He has no complaints and does not wear glasses.

   Examination Data:

   VA: OD 20/15
   OS 20/100; no improvement with pinhole

   Comment: During examination, this patient revealed that he has been aware since childhood that his left eye was a so-called lazy eye—in other words, that he suffered from amblyopia. Referral is not indicated since the cause of decreased vision is established and since progressive loss is not occurring. Note that this healthy individual has better than 20/20 acuity in his right eye.

4. A fifty-year-old man visits your office because he noted decreased visual acuity in the right eye the preceding day, while accidentally occluding his left eye. Two years ago, when his present glasses were prescribed, his vision was equal in both eyes.

Examination Data:

VA: OD 20/50; no improvement with pinhole
     OS 20/20

Ophthalmoscopy: no abnormalities detected

Comment: This patient has an unexplained loss of vision of unknown duration in one eye. An unexplained decrease in vision in one or both eyes requires referral to an ophthalmologist, since it may indicate occult disease of the eyes or central nervous system that is not detectable by examination methods available to the primary care physician. In this case, the patient's decreased vision was due to a macular disturbance detectable only by advanced methods of examination (e.g., special lenses and fluorescein angiography).

Annotated References

1. Gittinger JW Jr: *Ophthalmology: A Clinical Introduction.* Boston, Little, Brown & Co, 1984.

    Chapter 1 (Ocular History and Examination) covers the eye examination in this excellent introductory text for medical students.

2. Miller D: *Ophthalmology: The Essentials.* New York, Wiley & Sons, 1979.

    This book is extremely readable and geared particularly for medical students. Chapter 1 (Structure and Function of the Eye) and Chapter 2 (Testing) contain interesting discussions and useful illustrations.

3. Pavan-Langston D: *Manual of Ocular Diagnosis and Therapy* (ed 2). Boston, Little, Brown & Co, 1985.

    Chapter 1 (Ocular Examination Techniques and Diagnostic Tests) of this spiral manual covers the full gamut of techniques, including those which would only be used by an ophthalmologist.

4. Scheie HG, Albert DM: *Textbook of Ophthalmology* (ed 9). Philadelphia, WB Saunders Co, 1977.

    This comprehensive text covers in detail anatomy (Chapter 1), physiology (Chapter 5), symptoms of eye disease (Chapter 7), and examination techniques (Chapter 8).

5. Vaughan D, Asbury T: *General Ophthalmology* (ed 11). Los Altos, Lange Medical Publications, 1986.

    This is a useful and popular textbook for medical students, nonophthalmic physicians, and ophthalmology residents. Chapter 1 (Anatomy) contains good anatomical illustrations and Chapters 3 (Examination) and 4 (Ophthalmoscopic Examination) contain additional information on ophthalmic instruments and examination techniques.

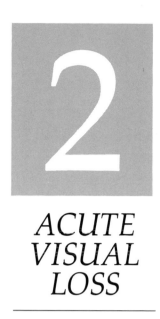

ACUTE VISUAL LOSS

Objectives

As a primary care physician, you should be able to evaluate a patient complaining of acute visual loss and construct a differential diagnosis, recognizing those situations where urgent action is necessary.

To achieve these objectives you should learn:

- What questions to ask the patient.
- How to distinguish acute visual loss caused by opacity of the media from that caused by retinal and optic nerve disease, using a penlight and ophthalmoscope.

Relevance

For most people, sudden blindness is a paradigm of disaster. Certainly, the patient who has experienced sudden loss of vision is understandably anxious and upset. The importance of identifying the cause of the visual loss and the potential treatment alternatives is apparent.

Basic Information

History

Important questions to ask in the event of sudden visual loss include:

- Is visual loss transient or persistent?

- Is visual loss monocular or binocular?
- What was the tempo? Did visual loss occur abruptly, or did it develop over hours, days, or weeks?
- What is the patient's age and medical condition?
- Did the patient have documented normal vision in the past?

Ocular Examination

Visual acuity. The first thing to be determined is the visual acuity, with best correction, in each eye. Normal acuity does not assure that significant vision has not been lost, since the entire visual field, including peripheral vision, must be considered. For instance, a patient who has lost all of the peripheral vision to one side—a homonymous hemianopia—generally has normal visual acuity.

Pupillary reactions. The reaction of the pupils to light is very useful in the evaluation of visual loss, especially when that reaction is asymmetrical between the two eyes. In what is called the swinging flashlight test, a bright light is moved from one eye to the other, and the pupillary reactions are observed. Both pupils should constrict as light falls upon either of them. The pupillary reaction of the eye upon which the light is directed is the more easily observed, but normally both pupils remain the same size. When the flashlight, or penlight, is moved from one eye to the other, the pupils dilate as the penlight beam crosses the nose. When the beam reaches the second eye, the now slightly dilated pupils again constrict.

When there is a lesion in the retina or the optic nerve of one eye, the brain stem centers controlling pupillary size perceive the light as being brighter in the normal eye. Thus, when the penlight beam is moved from the normal eye to the abnormal eye, the pupil of the abnormal eye may continue to dilate. This is the positive swinging flashlight test, which indicates a relative afferent pupillary defect, sometimes known as the Marcus Gunn pupil. The presence or absence of a relative afferent pupillary defect is often an important piece of information in the evaluation of monocular visual loss. *(For further information on pupillary pathways, see Chapter 7, Neuro-Ophthalmology.)*

Ophthalmoscopy. This is probably the most important examination technique in the evaluation of visual loss, because it allows visualization of the fundus and an assessment of the clarity of the refractive media.

Other Tests

- Slit-lamp examination will reveal the presence of any corneal or lenticular opacities or irregularities responsible for decreased vision.
- The use of tonometry to measure intraocular pressure provides an important clue about the presence or absence of glaucoma.

Differential Diagnosis

Opacity of the Media

The refractive medium of the eye—through which light must pass to reach the retina—is made up of the cornea, anterior chamber, lens, and vitreous. Usually, media opacities do not produce relative afferent pupillary defects; however, any irregularity or opacity in the media reduces vision. Acute visual loss may result from conditions that cause rapid changes in the transparency of these tissues.

Corneal edema. One cause of sudden opacification of the cornea is corneal edema. The most common cause of corneal edema is increased intraocular pressure. Visual loss accompanying an attack of angle-closure glaucoma is largely the result of corneal edema. Corneal edema is recognized by a dulling of the normally crisp reflection of incident light off the cornea. The cornea, crystal clear when healthy, takes on a ground glass appearance. Chronic damage to the corneal endothelium by dystrophies or following cataract surgery produces corneal edema, but the visual loss has a gradual onset. Acute infection by herpes simplex may mimic corneal edema *(see Chapter 4, Red Eye)*.

Hyphema. Blood in the anterior chamber is known as a hyphema *(see Chapter 5, Injuries, Fig. 42)*. A complete hyphema allows the perception of light only. Lesser degrees of hyphema may not affect visual acuity. Most hyphemas are the direct consequence of blunt trauma to a normal eye; however, the presence of abnormal vessels—which occurs with tumors, diabetes, and chronic inflammation, all causes of neovascularization—predisposes to hyphemas. Abnormal vessels may develop around intraocular lenses, and small hyphemas presenting as sudden visual loss are one complication of lens implantation for cataracts.

Cataracts. Most cataracts develop slowly. The rare patient may interpret rapid progression of a cataract as sudden visual loss. Even in a patient with clear lenses, sudden changes in blood sugar or serum electrolytes can alter the hydration of the lens. These changes in lens hydration can result in large fluctuations in refractive error, which may be interpreted by the patient as visual loss. Actually, acuity is restored with simple refraction.

Vitreous hemorrhage. Bleeding into the vitreous reduces vision in the same way that hyphema does: in relation to the amount of opaque blood present and to its location. Large vitreous hemorrhages occur after trauma, and in diabetics with neovascularization. In addition, vitreous hemorrhage may accompany subarachnoid hemorrhage, and is one cause of visual loss from aneurysms. Vitreous hemorrhages may be difficult to appreciate when viewed with the ophthalmoscope, especially through an undilated pupil. If the red reflex cannot be seen, and yet the lens appears clear, vitreous hemorrhage should be suspected. Diagnosis can be confirmed by slit-lamp examination through a dilated pupil, which would make visible any blood behind the lens.

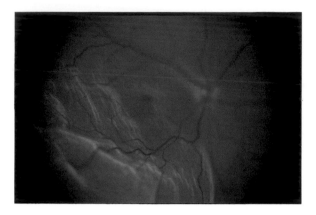

Fig. 6. Retinal detachment. A 60° panoramic view of the fundus reveals folds of retina extending into the macula inferotemporal to the disc. In this photograph, the focus is on the elevated retina, which renders the disc slightly out of focus.

Retinal Disease

Retinal detachments, macular disease, and vascular occlusions are all associated with sudden visual loss. However, acute visual loss may develop in any inflammatory process that affects the retina, including infectious chorioretinitis, vasculitides, and idiopathic inflammations. These conditions may be distinguished from other causes of acute visual loss by their ophthalmoscopic findings.

Retinal Detachments

Acute visual loss is a feature of extensive retinal detachments. Typically, the patient with a retinal detachment **(Fig. 6)** complains of flashing lights followed by large numbers of floaters, and then a shade over the vision in one eye. A detachment extensive enough to reduce visual acuity usually produces a relative afferent pupillary defect in the involved eye. The diagnosis is made by ophthalmoscopy through the dilated pupil. However, the findings may not be obvious, and ophthalmological consultation is indicated.

Macular Disease

Macular disease reduces visual acuity, but unless the disease is extensive, relative afferent pupillary defect may not be present. In a young person, the sudden onset of decreased vision and the perception of a spot in front

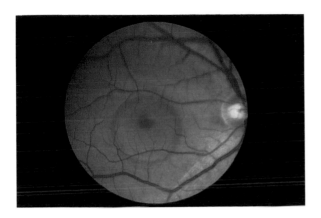

Fig. 7. Central serous choroidopathy. A dome of elevated sensory retina is seen in the macula.

of the eye (i.e., a positive scotoma) should raise the possibility of central serous choroidopathy **(Fig. 7)**. This condition is a serous elevation of the sensory retina in the region of the macula that appears as a clear dome on ophthalmoscopy. In an older person, sudden visual loss from macular disease is often an index of bleeding from a neovascular net formed as part of the process of senile macular degeneration *(see Chapter 3, Chronic Visual Loss)*. If this is preceded by metamorphopsia (i.e., a defect of central vision in which the shapes of objects appear distorted), the neovascularization may be identified and treated with laser before progression to significant visual loss occurs.

Vascular Occlusions

Vascular occlusions are a relatively common cause of sudden, severe visual loss. Permanent visual loss or other completed strokes may be preceded by periods of transient monocular visual loss, also called *amaurosis fugax,* or *fleeting blindness*. In a patient over the age of fifty years, the report of a period of visual loss in one eye lasting for several minutes should lead to investigation of the ipsilateral carotid circulation, looking for an atheroma, which may be the source of emboli that transiently interrupt blood flow to the retina. The evaluation and management of such patients raises complicated issues, and referral should be made to an ophthalmologist, neurologist, or vascular surgeon.

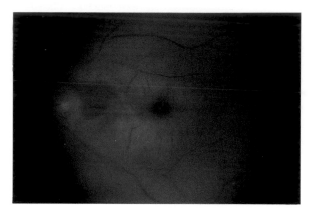

Fig. 8. Central retinal artery occlusion. The entire retina is opaque, except for the relatively thin area within the macula, producing the "cherry-red spot."

Central retinal artery occlusion. The prolonged interruption of retinal arterial blood flow causes permanent damage to the ganglion cells and other tissue elements. This is a central retinal artery occlusion **(Fig. 8)** and presents as sudden, painless, and often complete visual loss. The ophthalmoscopic appearance depends on how soon after the visual loss the fundus is visualized. Minutes to hours later, the only findings may be vascular stasis: narrowing of arterial and interruption of venous blood columns. The appearance of the venules is called "box-carring" because rows of corpuscles are separated by clear intervals.

Some hours after a central retinal artery occlusion, the inner layer of the retina swells and becomes opalescent. The loss of the normal transparency of the retina is most visible ophthalmoscopically, where the retina is thickest around the fovea. In the fovea itself, the inner layers are attenuated, and the edema of the perifoveal retina stands in contrast with the normal color of the fovea. This is the cause of the characteristic "cherry-red spot" of central retinal artery occlusion. A chronic cherry-red spot is also a feature of storage diseases, such as Tay-Sachs disease and some variants of Niemann-Pick disease, in which the ganglion cells become opalescent because of the deposition of intermediate metabolites.

The disc, which is supplied by other branches of the ophthalmic artery, does not swell unless the occlusion is in the ophthalmic or carotid artery, proximal to the origin of the central retinal artery. The peculiarities of the eye's vascular supply also explain the preservation of some vision in the presence of a complete central retinal artery occlusion. If part of the retina derives its blood supply from the choroidal circulation via a cilioretinal artery, its function is spared. Since cilioretinal arteries are relatively common anomalies, present in up to one fourth of all eyes, small islands of vision may be preserved after central retinal artery occlusion. If the territory of the cilioretinal artery includes both the macula and the disc, a visual acuity of 20/20 is possible, but there is severe loss of peripheral field. After a central retinal artery occlusion, the retinal edema slowly resolves, and the death of the ganglion cells and their axons leads to optic atrophy. Months later, the characteristic ophthalmoscopic appearance is a pale disc in a blind eye.

When the diagnosis of an acute central retinal artery occlusion is made, immediate treatment is warranted if there are still ophthalmoscopic signs of vascular stasis. This is a true ophthalmic emergency; restoration of blood flow may preserve vision if the occlusion is only a few hours old. Instances are reported where vision has returned after treatment of an occlusion that has been present for several days. In a blind eye there is little to lose by aggressive measures, and an ophthalmologist's advice should be obtained as quickly as possible.

The primary care physician might want simply to compress the eye with the heel of the hand, pressing firmly for ten seconds, and then releasing for ten seconds. The sudden rise and fall in intraocular pressure could serve to dislodge a small embolus in the central retinal artery, restoring circulation before the retinal tissues sustained irreversible damage. An ophthalmologist might employ more vigorous and invasive techniques, including retrobulbar injections of anesthetics and paracentesis of the anterior chamber.

Branch retinal artery occlusion. When only a branch of the central retinal artery is occluded, only part of the retina opacifies, and vision is only partially lost. Branch retinal artery occlusions are more likely to be the result of emboli than are central retinal artery occlusions, and a source should be sought. Because the visual acuity is usually normal in any eye with a branch retinal artery occlusion, vigorous treatment is not usually warranted.

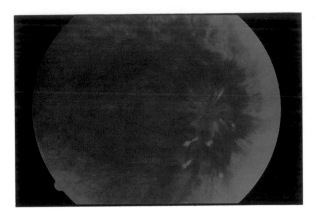

Fig. 9. Central retinal vein occlusion. Dilated and tortuous veins, flame-shaped hemorrhages, and cotton-wool spots characterize this condition.

Central retinal vein occlusion. The ophthalmoscopic picture of disc swelling, venous engorgement, cotton-wool spots, and diffuse retinal hemorrhages is called central retinal vein occlusion **(Fig. 9).** Visual loss may be severe, although the onset is generally subacute, unlike the dramatic sudden blindness of central retinal artery occlusion. The fundus picture is so striking that the description "blood and thunder" is sometimes applied. Despite its dramatic appearance, there is no generally accepted acute management, and a central retinal vein occlusion is not a true ophthalmic emergency.

Central retinal vein occlusion is most often encountered in older patients with hypertension and arteriosclerotic vascular disease. Carotid occlusion may produce a similar fundus picture. In rare cases, diseases that alter blood viscosity, such as polycythemia vera, sickle-cell disease, and lymphoma-leukemia, induce central retinal vein occlusions.

The acute hemorrhages and disc swelling resolve with time; however, they may be followed by the development of shunt vessels from the retinal to the choroidal circulation and ocular neovascularization. The patient with a central retinal vein occlusion needs a general medical evaluation and follow-up by an ophthalmologist, who may be able to prevent the late complication of neovascular glaucoma by laser photocoagulation of ischemic retina.

Optic Nerve Disease

Optic Neuritis

Optic neuritis is an inflammation of the optic nerve that is usually idiopathic but may be associated with multiple sclerosis in a significant number of cases. A relative afferent pupillary defect is a regular feature of optic neuritis. The prognosis for the return of vision after a single attack of optic neuritis is good. Some ophthalmologists use corticosteroids to treat patients with acute optic neuritis, and this does seem to speed recovery.

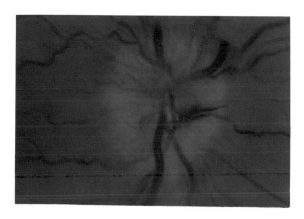

Fig. 10. Papillitis. The disc is swollen with hemorrhage. Note the similarity of appearance to ischemic optic neuropathy (see Fig. 12), except that in papillitis the disc is hyperemic rather than pale. When bilateral, papillitis is difficult to distinguish from papilledema ophthalmoscopically; however, visual loss is more marked in papillitis.

There is, however, no clear evidence that a course of steroids improves the eventual outcome of an attack of optic neuritis. Accordingly, other ophthalmologists and neurologists prefer not to treat the patient with acute optic neuritis, arguing that spontaneous resolution will ensue in weeks to months.

Retrobulbar Optic Neuritis

A young adult who presents with monocular loss of vision developing over hours to days and often accompanied by pain on movement of the eye, but who shows no abnormalities on ophthalmoscopic examination, probably has retrobulbar optic neuritis. The major differential factor in the diagnosis of retrobulbar optic neuritis is compressive optic neuropathy, which can present as acute visual loss. The pattern of visual field loss may point to a noninflammatory etiology, for example, by identifying visual field loss in the fellow eye. Computed tomography of the orbits and chiasmal region will identify most compressive lesions, which are potentially treatable with surgery.

Papillitis and Papilledema

Like retrobulbar optic neuritis, papillitis **(Fig. 10)** is a subgroup of optic neuritis. Specifically, papillitis is an inflammation of the optic disc, or papilla. Papilledema **(Fig. 11),** on the other hand, is an abnormal collection of fluid in the tissues of the optic disc. A classic distinction is made between papillitis and papilledema: In papillitis, the examiner doesn't see very much, and neither does the patient; whereas, in papilledema, the examiner and the patient see a lot.

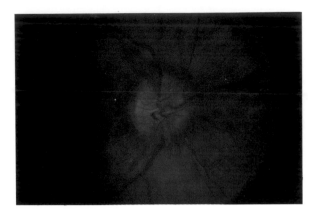

Fig. 11. Advanced papilledema. The optic disc is elevated and the margins are indistinct. There is microvascular congestion on the disc, the retinal veins are dilated, and numerous flame-shaped hemorrhages are present.

Like most maxims, this oversimplifies the situation, but it is true that disc swelling with visual loss points to papillitis; whereas, disc swelling with good vision points to papilledema. Some patients with acute papilledema complain of momentary blurring of vision, so-called transient obscurations of vision. Although chronic papilledema may lead to loss of vision, most patients with acute papilledema suffer only minor alterations in vision. This is in sharp contrast to patients with papillitis, most of whom experience significant visual loss.

Ischemic Optic Neuropathy

Swelling of the disc and visual loss in an older adult is likely to represent a vascular event rather than inflammation. Ischemic optic neuropathy **(Fig. 12)** is a vascular disorder that presents as a pale, swollen disc, often accompanied by splinter hemorrhages and visual loss. Many eyes with papillitis have poor central vision but good peripheral vision. This combination produces what is known as a *central scotoma* on visual field testing. In contrast to papillitis, visual loss due to ischemic optic neuropathy is often predominately in the superior or inferior field, a pattern known as *altitudinal.* Visual acuity is more likely to be reduced with papillitis than with ischemic optic neuropathy, but there are exceptions.

Giant-Cell (Temporal) Arteritis

The development of acute ischemic optic neuropathy in a patient over the age of sixty years raises the possibility of giant-cell, or temporal, arteritis. When this systemic arteritis is present, there are often associated complaints of malaise, limb girdle pain, scalp tenderness or discomfort when combing the hair, and a virtually pathognomonic pain in the jaws on chewing, termed *jaw claudication.*

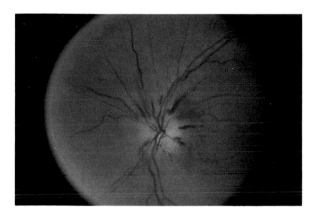

Fig. 12. Ischemic optic neuropathy. This figure shows pale swelling of the optic disc, with associated flame-shaped hemorrhages.

Even in an otherwise asymptomatic elderly patient who presents with ischemic optic neuropathy (or, for that matter, central retinal artery occlusion or an unexplained ophthalmoplegia), a sedimentation rate should be obtained immediately. Many elderly persons with giant-cell arteritis have markedly elevated sedimentation rates, to greater than 60 mm/hr. If the sedimentation rate is elevated or if there are other symptoms or signs of giant-cell arteritis, treatment with high-dose systemic steroids should be considered since this may preserve vision in the remaining eye and prevent vascular occlusions elsewhere that would cause stroke and myocardial infarction. Biopsy of the temporal artery may demonstrate pathological changes that confirm the diagnosis: giant cells, fragmentation of the elastica with surrounding chronic inflammation, and occlusion of the vessel.

If no systemic arteritis is demonstrated, there is no clear evidence that systemic steroids benefit patients with ischemic optic neuropathy, although some ophthalmologists still give short course treatment. Unfortunately, there is an approximately forty percent chance that the fellow eye will become involved with nonarteritic ischemic optic neuropathy, with or without treatment.

Trauma

Trauma is another potential cause of visual loss due to involvement of the optic nerve. Apparently, in a small number of cases, concussive head trauma shears the vascular supply to the optic nerve, producing blindness. There is no clear evidence that surgical intervention restores vision, but because the prognosis is so poor, surgery is sometimes undertaken.

Visual Pathway Disorders

Hemianopias. The cerebral visual pathways are susceptible to involvement by vascular events or tumors. In older persons, homonymous hemianopia is encountered regularly. This condition can be defined as loss of vision to one side as the result of occlusion of one of the posterior cerebral arteries, and infarction of the occipital lobe. Other vascular events occurring in the middle cerebral artery distribution also may produce hemianopias, but usually other neurological signs are prominent. Almost any patient who presents with a hemianopia warrants examination with cerebral computed tomography to localize and identify the cause.

Cortical blindness. Much rarer than an isolated hemianopia is extensive damage to the cerebral visual pathways resulting in the complete loss of vision. This condition is referred to variously as cortical, central, or cerebral blindness. Because the pathways serving the pupillary light reflex separate from those carrying visual information at the level of the optic tracts, a patient who is cortically blind has normal pupillary reactions. This finding, along with a normal ophthalmoscopic examination, helps make the diagnosis of cortical blindness. Most patients with cortical blindness either improve or expire due to severe neurological damage. Transient cortical blindness has been observed in children after subconcussive head trauma.

Functional Disorders

The adjective *functional* is used in preference to hysterical or malingering to describe visual loss without organic basis. Often the diagnosis is apparent because the examination produces results incompatible with organic blindness. For example, the patient who reports complete blindness in one eye and normal vision in the other, and yet has normal stereopsis and no relative afferent pupillary defect most likely has a functional disorder. In other patients, sophisticated ophthalmological examinations may be necessary in order to make an accurate diagnosis.

Acute Discovery of Chronic Visual Loss

It is surprising how many cases of chronic visual loss present as an acute discovery. Upon examination, a person given clear evidence of a chronic process may suddenly become aware of a visual deficit. Since the eyes usually function together, this sudden discovery of what is actually an ongoing problem is most likely to occur when the vision in one eye is normal. A person who claims acute visual loss in one eye and yet has advanced optic atrophy must have had a prolonged but unrecognized problem. In doubtful cases, it is desirable to obtain records of previous formal eye examinations before accepting visual loss as an acute event and proceeding with expensive or invasive workups.

Sample Problems

Case Analysis

1. A fifty-eight-year-old woman complains of a sudden shower of dust-like opacities floating before the vision of her right eye.

   Examination Data:

   Visual acuity: 20/20 each eye; dilated fundus examination normal.

   Diagnosis: Possible retinal tear, danger of retinal detachment.

   Management: Prompt ophthalmic consultation.

   Comment: A sudden shower of floaters may indicate red blood cells in the vitreous due to a retinal tear. Floaters may be visible to the patient but not to the ophthalmoscopist. Since the retina has no sensitivity to pain and is, in fact, limited to the sensation of light, the patient may report light flashes as the retina tears or detaches. Retinal tears usually are located in the far periphery of the retina and may easily elude detection. Symptoms alone indicate the need for referral.

2. A sixty-seven-year-old man experienced sudden loss of vision in the left eye three hours ago.

   Examination Data:

   Visual acuity: Right eye, 20/20; left eye, no light perception. The right pupil responds to light directly but not consensually. The left pupil responds to light consensually but not directly. Dilated fundus examination of the right eye is normal. The left eye shows white, opacified retina, cherry-red spot in the macula, and sluggish retinal circulation.

   Diagnosis: Central retinal artery occlusion.

   Management: You use the heel of your hand to apply pressure to the affected eye, pressing and releasing several times, in the hope that the induced alterations of intraocular pressure might dislodge an embolus. You seek ophthalmic consultation and undertake a prompt search for the cause of this vascular event.

   Comment: Since the retina is neural tissue and survives complete circulatory deprivation poorly, the prognosis for recovery of vision in the affected eye is not good. Probably most important is the detection of underlying disease (such as giant-cell arteritis) or a site of embolus formation (such as carotid atheroma) that might lead to future vascular occlusions.

Annotated References

1. Gutman FA: Evaluation of a patient with central retinal vein occlusion. *Ophthalmology* **90:**481–483, 1983.

   One of several articles in the same volume of this journal outlining the diagnosis, evaluation, and management of central retinal vein occlusions.

2. Hurwitz BJ, Heyman A, Wilkinson WE, et al: Comparison of amaurosis fugax and transient cerebral ischemia: A prospective clinical and arteriographic study. *Ann Neurol* **18:**698–704, 1985.

   This series of over three hundred patients with amaurosis fugax or cerebral transient ischemic attacks is part of a large literature on the subject, but one of the few prospective studies. Two-thirds of the middle-aged or elderly patients with amaurosis fugax had operable carotid lesions.

3. Jaeger EA: Venous obstructive disease of the retina, in Duane TD (ed): *Clinical Ophthalmology.* Philadelphia, Harper & Row, 1985, vol 3, ch 15.

   A chapter in an encyclopedic volume that reviews the subject of central retinal vein occlusions.

4. Miller NR: *Walsh & Hoyt's Clinical Neuro-Ophthalmology,* ed 4. Baltimore, Williams & Wilkins, 1982, vol 1.

   The second volume of this excellent three-volume set provides an extensive discussion of disorders of the optic nerve.

5. Ravits J, Seybold ME: Transient monocular visual loss from narrow-angle glaucoma. *Arch Neurol* **41:**991–993, 1984.

   Three patients with intermittent angle-closure had their transient visual loss attributed to other causes until glaucoma was considered.

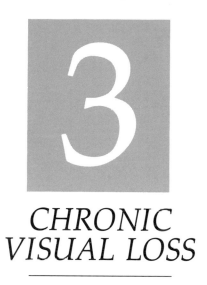

CHRONIC
VISUAL LOSS

Objectives

In an adult patient, you should be familiar with the major causes of chronic, slowly progressive visual loss, namely glaucoma, cataract, and macular degeneration, and be able to identify the basic characteristics of each. *(See also Chapter 8, Ocular Manifestations of Systemic Disease, for a discussion of diabetic retinopathy, another important cause of chronic visual loss.)* In addition, you should be able to measure the intraocular pressure with a Schiotz tonometer and to evaluate the nerve head, classifying it as normal, glaucomatous, or abnormal but nonglaucomatous. You should be able to evaluate macular function and appearance.

To achieve these objectives you should learn:

- To recognize those characteristics of the optic disc useful in determining whether a given disc is normal or abnormal.
- To demonstrate how a Schiotz tonometer functions, including the way in which it is used to measure intraocular pressure.
- To recognize a cataract and to determine its approximate potential effect on the patient's vision.
- To determine if a cataract is the only cause of a patient's visual decrease.
- To examine the macula with the ophthalmoscope.

PART 1. GLAUCOMA

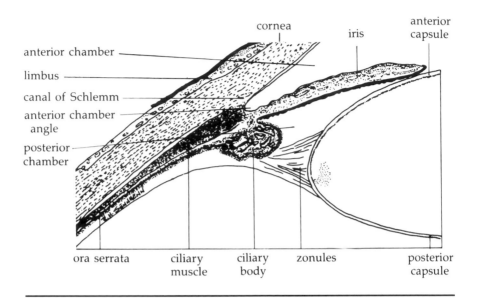

Illus. 3.1. Cross-section of anterior chamber angle and ciliary body

Relevance

Glaucoma is the third major cause of blindness in the United States, accounting for approximately twelve percent of all new cases of blindness each year. If glaucoma is detected early and treated medically or surgically, blindness can be prevented. Most patients with early glaucoma are asymptomatic. The great majority of patients lack pain, ocular inflammation, or halos (luminous or colored rings seen around lights). Much peripheral vision can be lost before the patient notices visual impairment.

Glaucoma is usually insidious because symptoms and noticeable visual field defects occur late in the disease. Visual field defects are characterized by arcuate-shaped scotomas and a silent contraction of the peripheral field, sparing the central vision until late in the disease process. Detection in the early asymptomatic stage requires an active effort. The early detection of glaucoma is important because glaucomatous blindness can usually be prevented if the disease is treated adequately and if treatment is begun in time.

Because glaucoma is a disease which involves elevated pressure in the eye, routine measurement of intraocular pressure is a means of screening for glaucoma. Prolonged elevated intraocular pressure can lead to optic nerve damage, therefore examination of the optic nerve is another way to detect glaucoma. Other disorders, such as a brain tumor, can also cause changes in the optic nerve, making the ability to recognize other abnormalities of the optic nerve important in and of itself.

Basic Information

Intraocular Pressure

Within the eye, there is a mechanism for the continuous production and drainage of fluid. This fluid is called aqueous humor and is produced by the ciliary body of the eye. Aqueous humor flows through the pupil into the anterior chamber, where it is drained through the trabecular meshwork to Schlemm's canal **(Illus. 3.1),** and onward to the venous system. Because there is some resistance to the flow of aqueous through the trabeculum and Schlemm's canal, a pressure is created in the eye. All eyes have an internal pressure.

The intraocular pressure is largely dependent on the ease of flow through the trabeculum and Schlemm's canal. The greater the resistance to flow, the higher the pressure in the eye. Although the eye contains several compartments within it, for purposes of pressure it can be considered a single closed space. Thus, the pressure exerted within the eye is equal over the entire wall of the eye.

Most normal eyes have an intraocular pressure of 21.5 mm Hg or less. This fact is valuable in screening for glaucoma. In the common, insidious form of glaucoma, the chamber angle remains open. Accordingly, this form of glaucoma is called open-angle glaucoma. In rare instances, the trabeculum can become suddenly and completely occluded by iris tissue. This causes an abrupt rise in intraocular pressure known as acute angle-closure glaucoma *(see Chapter 4, Red Eye, Fig. 22)* and constitutes an ocular emergency. The abrupt rise in pressure causes symptoms not found in the insidious form of glaucoma, including pain, nausea, and the visualization of colored halos or rainbows around light. Examination of the eye during an acute attack of angle closure usually reveals a red, teary eye with a hazy cornea and a fixed, mid-dilated pupil. The eye usually feels extremely firm to palpation.

Optic Nerve

The optic nerve is composed of over 1.2 million nerve fibers. These nerve fibers originate in the ganglion cells of the retina, gather in a bundle as the optic nerve, and carry visual information to the brain. An interruption of these nerve fibers will result in damage to vision.

The optic nerve can be seen at its origin by using the ophthalmoscope. At the point of origin, the nerve is called the optic disc. The optic disc often has a small depression in it called the cup of the optic disc. The size of the cup in normal eyes can vary with the individual.

Relationship of Intraocular Pressure and the Optic Nerve

Intraocular pressure is exerted on all walls of the eye, including the optic nerve and its blood vessels. The optic nerve is supplied with blood via branches of the ophthalmic artery, itself a branch of the internal carotid artery. If pressure in the eye is too high, the result may be that blood is prevented from adequately perfusing the optic nerve. If prolonged, this deficiency can cause damage to the nerve.

Damage to the optic nerve then results in visual field loss. Such loss is selective, but can become severe and even total over time. Detection of glaucomatous visual loss is accomplished by visual field testing. Visual acuity usually does not suffer initially. Measurement of intraocular pressure and evaluation of optic nerve appearance can detect potential and actual damage so that proper evaluation and treatment can be initiated.

Measurement of Intraocular Pressure

Palpation can only detect very hard and very soft eyes; it is totally unreliable in the range of the most common glaucomatous pressures. Intraocular pressure is best measured via tonometry, which may be performed in several ways. Indentation, or Schiotz, tonometry is the most common method. The technique is easy to perform, takes only a minute or two, and is painless and safe for the patient. *(Refer to Chapter 1, The Eye Examination, for the technique of Schiotz tonometry.)*

When and How to Examine

Tonometry and ophthalmoscopy should be part of every comprehensive eye examination. Information on Schiotz tonometry and the use of the direct ophthalmoscope can be found in *Chapter 1, The Eye Examination.* Particular attention should be given to (1) patients who are predisposed, for example, the diabetic patient; (2) patients with a family history of glaucoma; and (3) patients over forty years of age, since the incidence of glaucoma increases with age.

How to Interpret an Abnormal Optic Disc

The appearance of the optic disc can be described generally in terms of its color and the size of its physiologic cup **(Fig. 13)**. One commonly used descriptor of the optic disc is the ratio of the horizontal diameter of the cup to that of the disc, or the cup disc ratio **(Fig. 14)**. The size of the cup changes little with aging and must be distinguished from acquired glaucomatous cupping.

The color of the optic nerve can be important in determining atrophy of the optic nerve due to glaucoma or other causes. Temporal pallor of the optic nerve **(Fig. 15)** can occur as a result of diseases that damage the nerve fibers, such as brain tumors or optic nerve inflammation, or in conjunction with glaucomatous cupping. A large cup **(Fig. 16)** should be suspected if central pallor of the disc is prominent. Because the cup is a depressed area of the disc, retinal vessels passing over the disc are seen to bend at the edge of the cup. This is also a useful sign in evaluating the size of the cup. Thus, both color and vessel displacement should be

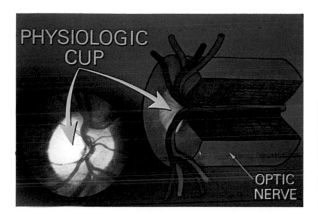

Fig. 13. Physiologic cup. This figure demonstrates the location of the physiologic cup relative to the optic disc. (The illuminated circle represents the field of view of the direct ophthalmoscope.)

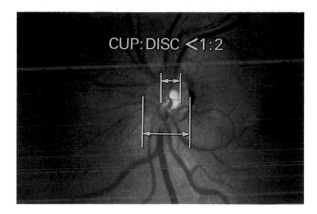

Fig. 14. Cup disc ratio. The cup disc ratio shown here is 0.4; the cup is slightly less than one half the diameter of the disc.

evaluated in determining the size of the cup. A cup larger than one half the size of the disc—a cup disc ratio greater than 0.5—is suspicious. The larger the cup, the greater the possibility of a glaucomatous optic nerve.

The optic discs nearly always appear symmetrical between the two eyes. Discs which exhibit asymmetry of the cup disc ratios should arouse suspicion. In some cases, there may be edema of the optic disc. This is called papilledema when caused by elevated intracranial pressure, and the cup may be reduced or obliterated. *(For a figure of advanced papilledema, see Chapter 2, Acute Visual Loss, Fig. 11.)*

An ophthalmologist evaluating a patient with suspected glaucoma will usually perform perimetry to formally evaluate the visual field. In addition, the anterior chamber angle structures can be visualized using a contact lens on the topically anesthetized cornea. This technique is called gonioscopy.

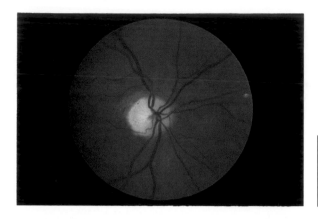

Fig. 15. Temporal pallor of the optic nerve. Diseases that damage the optic nerve fibers may result in temporal pallor of the optic nerve, as shown here.

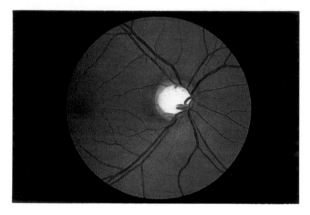

Fig. 16. Large physiologic cup. The horizontal cup disc ratio of the relatively large cup shown here is 0.8. Cupping is very apparent at the point at which the vessels disappear over the edge of the intact rim.

Management or Referral

Any patient who has one or more of the following conditions should be referred to an ophthalmologist:

- intraocular pressure over 21.5 mm Hg (i.e., a Schiotz reading of 3.5 units or less with a plunger load of 5.5 gm);
- intraocular pressure not elevated, but a difference of 5 mm Hg or more (i.e., 2 Schiotz scale units) exists between the two eyes;
- an optic cup diameter greater than one half of the disc diameter (i.e., cup disc ratio of 0.6 or greater);
- one cup is significantly larger than that of the fellow eye;
- a family history of glaucoma.

A patient with symptoms of acute glaucoma should be referred immediately.

PART 2. CATARACT

Relevance

Cataract may occur as a congenital and/or genetic anomaly, as a result of various diseases, or with increasing age. Some degree of cataract formation is to be expected in all persons over age seventy years. In fact, age-related ("senile") cataract occurs in sixty-five percent of people in their sixties and in over ninety-five percent of those over sixty-five years of age.

Cataract is the most common cause of decreased vision (not correctable with glasses) in the United States. However, it is one of the most successfully treated conditions in all of surgery. Approximately one million cataract extractions are done each year in the United States. Extraction usually leads to complete visual rehabilitation.

It is important to be certain that visual loss is explained fully by cataract and not by other causes of visual loss, such as glaucoma, macular degeneration, or diabetic retinopathy. Cataract may coexist with these conditions, making assessment more difficult.

Basic Information

Lens

The lens focuses a clear image on the retina. The crystalline lens is suspended by thin filamentous zonules from the ciliary body between the iris anteriorly and the vitreous humor posteriorly. Contraction of the ciliary muscle permits focusing of the lens. The lens is enclosed in a capsule of transparent elastic basement membrane. There is a single anterior layer of cuboidal epithelium inside of this capsule. This capsule encloses the cortex and the nucleus of the lens. The lens has no innervation or blood supply. Nourishment comes from the aqueous and vitreous.

The normal lens continues to grow throughout life. The epithelial cells continue to produce new cortical lens fibers, yielding a slow increase in size, weight, and density over the years. The normal lens consists of thirty-five percent protein by mass. The percentage of insoluble protein increases as the lens ages and as a cataract develops.

Cataract

A cataract is any opacity or discoloration of the lens, whether a small local opacity or the complete loss of transparency. Clinically, the term "cataract" is reserved for opacities that affect visual acuity, since many normal lenses may have small, visually insignificant opacities.

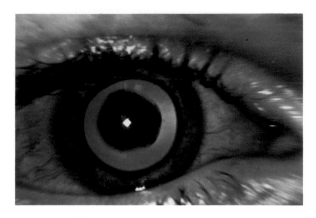

Fig. 17. Immature cataract. The nucleus of this lens is opaque (nuclear cataract), while the cortical layers remain clear. The opacity appears as a dark shadow against the red reflex. This particular cataract, which is congenital, will obstruct vision more when the pupil is small than when it is dilated as shown here.

Types of Cataracts

A cataract is described in terms of the zones of the lens involved in the opacity. These zones of opacity may be subcapsular, cortical, or nuclear, and may be anterior or posterior in location. In addition to opacification of the nucleus and cortex, there may be a yellow or amber color change to the lens. A cataract also can be described in terms of its stage of development. A cataract with clear cortex remaining is immature **(Fig. 17).** A mature cataract **(Fig. 18)** has a totally opacified cortex.

The most common cause of cataract is age-related change. Other etiological factors include trauma, inflammation, metabolic and nutritional defects, and radiation damage. Cataracts may develop very slowly over the years or may progress rapidly, depending on the etiology and type of cataract.

Symptomatology of Cataract

The patient may first notice image blur as the lens loses its ability to resolve separate and distinct objects. The patient is first aware of a disturbance of vision, then a diminution, and finally a failure of vision. The degree of disability caused by a cataract is dependent on the size and location of the opacity. Axial opacities—affecting the nucleus or central subcapsular areas **(see Fig. 17)**—cause much more trouble than peripheral opacities.

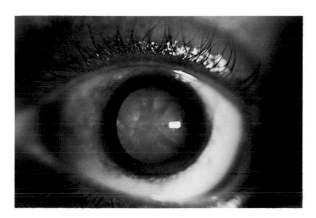

Fig. 18. Mature cataract. A cataract is called mature when the lens is totally opacified. A red reflex cannot be obtained; the pupil appears white. The radial spokes in this figure reflect variations in density of the radially arranged fibers in the cortical layers of the lens. Light still reaching the retina is totally diffused and will allow the perception of light but not form.

The patient with nuclear sclerosis may develop increasing lenticular (i.e., referring to the crystalline lens) myopia because of the increased refractive power of the denser nucleus. As the size of the cataract increases, the patient becomes progressively more myopic. The patient may find that he can read without the glasses he usually requires. This phenomenon is often called "second sight." The patient may note monocular double or multiple images. This is due to irregular refraction within the lens.

Patients with anterior or posterior subcapsular cataracts may note a relatively rapid decrease in vision. Subcapsular cataracts produce visual impairment with glare as well as image blur and distortion. This type of cataract is frequently associated with metabolic causes such as diabetes mellitus and corticosteroid use.

With enough time, all cataracts will lead to a generalized impairment of vision. The degree of impairment may vary from day to day. With yellowing of the lens nucleus, objects will appear browner or yellower to the patient than they actually are.

When to Examine

A patient with decreasing vision requires examination to determine the cause of the visual decrease. In testing, it is important to be able to demonstrate that the retina and optic nerve are healthy and that the visual decrease is due to lens changes only or primarily.

If the lens is densely cataractous, the ophthalmoscope will not provide a view of the fundus through the opacity, and other conditions cannot be ruled out. In this situation, the risk of overlooking other pathology exists, as does the risk of performing surgery for cataract without the assurance that vision loss is due primarily to lens changes.

In order to detect fundus changes early, ophthalmoscopic examination should be part of every physical examination. Special attention is given to the macula when a patient reports difficulty with near work, blurred vision, or metamorphopsia (i.e., a wavy distortion of central vision).

How to Examine and Interpreting the Findings

The following examination methods are particularly helpful in assessing a cataract.

- *Visual acuity measurement.* The first step in any evaluation of visual decrease is the measurement of visual acuity. Refer to *Chapter 1, The Eye Examination,* for details.

- *Examination of pupillary responses. Chapter 7, Neuro-Ophthalmology,* describes how to perform a basic pupillary examination and provides details on the neurological implications of pupillary responses.

- *Ophthalmoscopic examination.* The direct ophthalmoscope is helpful in the evaluation of cataracts. The examiner's view into the eye should be about the same as the patient's visual acuity; that is, the cataract should affect the physician's view into the eye to about the same extent as it does the patient's view out.

  The early cataract is not visible to the unaided eye. As the cataract becomes denser, it may appear as a white pupil, or leukocoria. The lens can be evaluated with the ophthalmoscope using a plus lens setting. The lens opacification will appear black against the red reflex of the retina. An ophthalmologist would routinely perform a slit-lamp examination, which provides a magnified stereoscopic view of the lens and other anterior segment structures.

Management or Referral

The decision to refer the patient with cataract should be based in part on whether or not the cataract keeps the patient from doing what he wants to do. If a cataract interferes with a patient's daily pattern of living, that patient may benefit from cataract extraction. It is important not to assign all visual loss to cataract when other, more serious causes of visual loss may be overlooked. If you can't "see in" clearly enough to evaluate the retina or optic nerve, the patient should always be referred to an ophthalmologist.

PART 3. MACULAR DEGENERATION

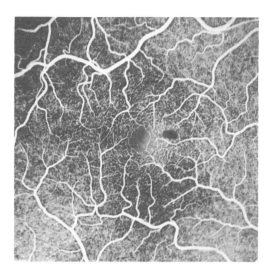

Photo 3.1. Central macula. The central macula is avascular, as demonstrated in this fundus fluorescein angiogram. The capillary-free zone identifies the foveal region. A small hemorrhage is made more visible against the fluorescein-enhanced background.

Relevance

In the United States, age-related macular degeneration is the leading cause of legal blindness in patients over sixty-five years of age. Because certain types of macular degeneration are treated effectively with laser, it is important to recognize this entity and refer for appropriate care. It is important to distinguish between the possible causes of visual loss, whether cataract (surgically correctable), glaucoma (medically or surgically treatable), or macular degeneration (potentially laser treatable).

Basic Information

Macular Anatomy

The macula is an oval area situated about two disc diameters temporal to and slightly below the optic disc *(see Chapter 1, The Eye Examination, Fig. 2, for figure of the normal fundus)*. The macula is composed of both rods and cones and is the area responsible for detailed, fine central vision. The central macula **(Photo 3.1)** is avascular and appears to be darker than the surrounding retina. The fovea is an oval depression in the center of the macula. Here, there is a high density of cones but no rods present. The central depression of the fovea may act as a concave mirror during ophthalmoscopy, producing a light reflection (i.e., foveal reflex).

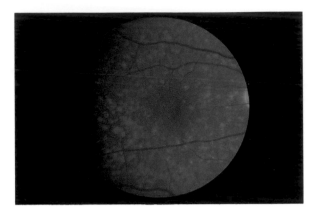

Fig. 19. Drusen. Distinct yellow-white lesions may be seen in the posterior pole surrounding the macular area. Although acuity may be normal initially, these lesions can lead to significant visual loss if the central macula becomes involved.

Age-Related Macular Changes

Macular changes due to age include drusen, degenerative changes in the retinal pigment epithelium, and subretinal neovascular membranes.

Drusen. Drusen are hyaline nodules (or colloid bodies) deposited in Bruch's membrane, which separates the inner choroidal vessels from the retinal pigment epithelium. These drusen may be small and discrete **(Fig. 19)** or larger, with irregular shapes and indistinct edges **(Fig. 20).** Patients with drusen alone will tend to have normal or near normal visual acuity with minimal metamorphopsia. Drusen may be seen with increasing age, during retinal or choroidal degeneration in disease states, and as a primary dystrophy.

Retinal pigment epithelial degenerative changes may occur with or without drusen. These degenerative changes are manifested as clumps of hyperpigmentation and/or depigmented atrophic areas **(Fig. 21).** The effect on visual acuity is variable.

Subretinal neovascular membranes. Twenty percent of eyes with age-related macular degeneration develop subretinal neovascularization. The extension of vessels from the choriocapillaries into the subpigment epithelial space and eventually into the subretinal space means that a defect has developed in Bruch's membrane.

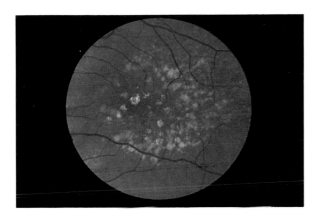

Fig. 20. Prominent drusen. This figure shows an advanced case; the drusen are exceptionally large and prominent, with a few areas of calcification.

The subretinal neovascular net may be associated with subretinal hemorrhage, fibrosis, pigment epithelial degeneration, and photoreceptor atrophy. A hemorrhage may result in acute visual loss (*see Chapter 2, Acute Visual Loss*). The larger the membrane is and the closer to the center of the fovea, the worse the prognosis is for good central vision.

Fluorescein angiography may be necessary to identify neovascularization and is mandatory before considering laser treatment. In this special technique utilized by ophthalmologists, intravenous injection of fluorescein dye will help demonstrate the retinal and choroidal vasculature. Unlike competent retinal veins and arteries, new vessels can be identified because they leak fluorescein dye. In addition, retinal pigment epithelium acts as a physical and optical barrier to fluorescein, and thus angiography facilitates identification of pigment epithelial defects.

Compare **Fig. 21,** a fundus photograph depicting subretinal hemorrhage and other age-related changes with **Photo 3.2,** a fundus fluorescein angiogram of the same eye which reveals neovascularization associated with the hemorrhage. These figures demonstrate both atrophy and neovascularization. In addition to age, other causes of chronic maculopathy include heredity and metabolic changes.

Age-related changes are almost totally confined to the posterior pole of the eye. Thus, the patient with macular degeneration may have very poor central vision, but will tend to retain functional, or "getting about," vision. Visual aids, such as high plus magnifiers and telescopic devices, may be able to help the patient.

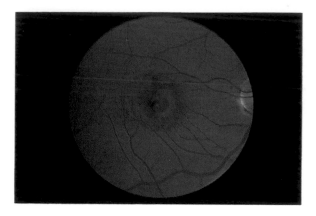

Fig. 21. Subretinal hemorrhage. Age-related macular changes often include subretinal hemorrhage, fibrosis, and pigment epithelial degeneration, as shown in this fundus photograph.

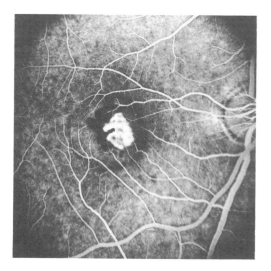

Photo 3.2. Neovascular net. This fluorescein angiogram of the same fundus shown in Fig. 21 reveals a subretinal neovascular net, responsible for the subretinal hemorrhage seen in that figure. In this angiogram, the net appears as a white, irregular area of fluorescein leakage.

When to Examine

Any patient with decreasing vision requires examination to determine the cause of the visual decrease. In assessing a patient with decreased or distorted central vision, every effort should be made to visualize the macula with the ophthalmoscope. Of course, opacities in the cornea, lens, or vitreous may preclude an adequate view of the macula.

How to Examine

The following techniques are especially helpful in evaluating macular degeneration as the cause of visual decrease or major changes in vision.

- *Visual acuity measurement.* Refer to *Chapter 1, The Eye Examination,* for the measurement of visual acuity.

- *Amsler grid testing.* Amsler grid testing **(Photo 3.3)** is a method of evaluating the function of the macula. The test is carried out by having the patient look with one eye at a time at a central spot on a page with horizontal and vertical parallel lines making up a square grid pattern. This grid pattern is usually printed in white against a black background. The patient is asked to note irregularities in the lines. Irregularities may be reported as lines that are wavy, seem to bow or bend, or appear gray or fuzzy, or that are absent in certain areas of the grid, indicating a scotoma.

  The straight line, right angle, and square are geometric figures in which the eye can distinguish distortions most easily. With the chart held at a normal reading distance of 30 centimeters from the eye, the Amsler grid measures 10 degrees on each side of fixation. This allows for an evaluation of 5.36 millimeters in all directions from the center of the macula (i.e., the fovea). Thus, the entire macula is evaluated with this examination.

- *Ophthalmoscopic examination.* The macular area is studied with the direct ophthalmoscope. Sometimes it is helpful to have the patient look directly into the light of the instrument. Dilation of the pupil may be necessary for adequate visualization.

- *Additional studies.* The ophthalmologist may elect to carry out special studies to better evaluate the macula and macular function. Studies such as stereoscopic slit-lamp examination and fluorescein angiography may be necessary to determine pathologic changes.

How to Interpret an Abnormal Macula

The appearance of the macula often does not accurately predict the visual acuity. The macula may look more or less involved than the vision indicates. The presence of drusen, areas of decreased and/or increased pigmentation, and the presence of hemorrhage or neovascularization are all important signs to check for in an examination of the macula. The absence of the foveal reflex and a mottled appearance of the underlying retinal pigment epithelium are among the early signs of macular disease.

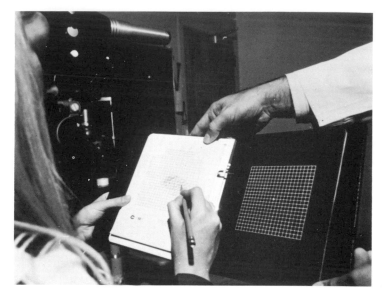

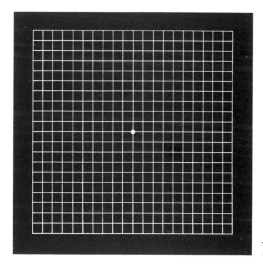

Photo 3.3. Amsler grid testing. (A) In this photograph, the patient indicates the nature and location of her central field defect by sketching what she perceives on the Amsler grid. (B) Shown here is the typical grid pattern of white lines against a black background.

Management or Referral

Any patient who has one or more of the following should be referred to an ophthalmologist:

- a recent onset of decreased clarity of vision;
- a recent onset of metamorphopsia, or distortion of central vision;
- a recent onset of a scotoma, or blind spot.

In addition, patients with any ophthalmoscopic abnormalities in the appearance of the macula, such as drusen, degenerative changes in the retinal pigment epithelium, or subretinal neovascular membranes, should be referred.

Sample Problems

Multiple Choice

1. During a thorough physical examination of a thirty-eight-year old male patient, you record intraocular pressures of 20 mm Hg in the right eye and 24 mm Hg in the left eye. Based on these findings, which of the following represents a reasonable course of action on your part?

    (a) Explain to the patient that he has glaucoma and that you want to recheck his intraocular pressures in three months.

    (b) Evaluate the optic discs carefully and, if they are normal, recheck the patient in six to twelve months.

    (c) Refer the patient to an ophthalmologist.

    (d) Inquire about a family history of glaucoma and, if there is none, reassure the patient that his intraocular pressures are probably in the upper range of normal.

    Answer: Choice (c). Elevated intraocular pressure alone is not a definite indication of glaucoma. It would be correct to tell this patient that his intraocular pressure is slightly elevated on this one occasion. In tonometry screening, it is best to determine the pressure and act accordingly rather than make decisions regarding a definitive diagnosis of glaucoma and a decision on management. Thus, the correct approach in this case is to refer the patient to an ophthalmologist since pressures of 22 mm Hg or higher are statistically abnormal. The ophthalmologist may decide merely to follow the patient without treatment, but this should be left to the ophthalmologist.

    It is good to know whether the optic discs are normal, but once you find an elevated pressure, your next move should be referral. On the other hand, in situations where you find a normal pressure but questionable optic discs, it is good to remember that glaucoma still could exist and that referral still may be indicated. Finally, although glaucoma has some hereditary aspects, this should have no bearing in a case in which you find elevated pressure. However, should you have a patient with a strong positive family history of glaucoma, it may be wise to suggest that the patient obtain an ophthalmologist's evaluation despite your finding normal pressures.

2. Your seventy-five-year-old neighbor is visiting your house. He says that your pictures and door jambs don't seem straight. He tells you that his vision isn't quite as sharp as it used to be and that lines seem to weave and bow. What do you think is going on and what do you advise?

   (a) Tell him that the person who hung your pictures could never get anything straight and ignore his opinion.

   (b) Tell him you will straighten your pictures.

   (c) Tell him that he may have some age-related macular changes and should seek consultation because, if there is evidence of subretinal neovascularization, he may benefit from early laser treatment.

   Answer: Choice (c). A patient with metamorphopsia may have drusen in the macula only and not be a candidate for laser treatment, but twenty percent of eyes with age-related macular degeneration develop subretinal neovascularization. Clinical studies have indicated that argon laser photocoagulation of subretinal neovascular membranes which are not too close to the fovea significantly reduce the central visual loss.

3. A retired patient of yours is developing nuclear sclerosis, and his visual acuity has decreased to OD 20/30 (right eye) and OS 20/40 (left eye). The only time his vision bothers him is in a dark restaurant, where he has some difficulty reading the menu. Friends have told him about a doctor who will operate with laser to remove his cataract without risk and who will do it for "free." He asks your advice. What do you tell him?

   (a) If it's free and he really is a doctor, then go ahead.

   (b) Tell him that laser is not used to remove cataracts, but he should go ahead anyway.

   (c) Advise that (1) the indications to remove a cataract are if it endangers the health of the eye or keeps the patient from doing what he needs and wants to do; (2) lasers are not used to remove cataracts, but this misconception may be presented; and (3) no surgery is free or without risk. The disability of decreased vision must warrant the risks inherent in surgery.

   Answer: Choice (c) is, of course, the appropriate response.

Annotated References

Glaucoma

1. Duane TD, Jaeger EA (eds): *Clinical Ophthalmology*. Philadelphia, Harper & Row, 1985, vol 3.

   One of several volumes in this annually updated set, this text provides a source of information on contemporary concepts about the glaucomas and their treatment. Both basic and sophisticated information are available in this volume.

2. Duke-Elder S (ed): Diseases of the lens & vitreous: Glaucoma & hypotony, in *System of Ophthalmology.* St. Louis, CV Mosby Co, 1969, vol 11.

   Volume 11 in this multiple-volume set is an encyclopedia of basic information on the glaucomas. It also covers in detail the evolution of our knowledge of glaucoma and the individuals involved in that process.

3. Epstein DL: *Chandler and Grant's Glaucoma,* ed 3. Philadelphia, Lea & Febiger, 1986.

   An excellent reference covering current medical and surgical therapies of the glaucomas. Special types of glaucoma are also covered.

Cataract

4. Duane TD, Jaeger EA (eds): *Clinical Ophthalmology.* Philadelphia, Harper & Row, 1985, vol 1.

   Provides basic background material and up-to-date information on cataracts, their impact on vision, and their management.

5. Duke-Elder S (ed): Diseases of the retina, in *System of Ophthalmology.* St. Louis, CV Mosby Co, 1967, vol 10.

   Offers an extensive historical review of cataracts. Emphasis is on associated medical conditions and varieties of cataract rather than on surgical management.

6. Jaffe NS: *Cataract Surgery and Its Complications,* ed 4. St. Louis, Mo, CV Mosby Co, 1984.

   An excellent text covering the contemporary methods of surgical management of cataracts and the complications associated with this surgery.

Macular Degeneration

7. Duane TD, Jaeger EA (eds): *Clinical Ophthalmology.* Philadelphia, Harper & Row, 1985, vol 3.

   Volume 3 in this multiple-volume set covers glaucoma and the retina. Because the set is updated annually, this text offers current information on our knowledge of macular degeneration.

8. Duke-Elder S (ed): Diseases of the uveal tract, in *System of Ophthalmology.* St. Louis, CV Mosby Co, 1966, vol 9.

   Readily available in all medical school and ophthalmology libraries, this set is a valuable reference tool. Volume 9 provides an attention to detail that should be of assistance to students seeking further information on macular degeneration.

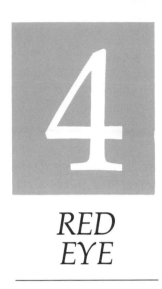

RED
EYE

Objective

In evaluating a patient with a red eye, you should be able to determine whether the disorder requires the prompt attention of an ophthalmologist or if you, as a primary care physician, can appropriately treat it.

To achieve this objective you should learn:

- To perform the nine diagnostic steps described under *How to Examine*.
- To recognize the danger signs discussed under *Interpreting the Findings*.
- To describe the serious complications of prolonged use of topical anesthetic drops and of corticosteroids discussed under *Therapeutic Warnings*.
- To describe the treatment for those cases the primary care physician can treat and to recognize the more serious problems which should be referred, covered under *Management or Referral*.

Relevance

A primary care physician frequently encounters patients who complain of a red eye. The condition causing the red eye is often a simple disorder such as a subconjunctival hemorrhage or an infectious conjunctivitis. These conditions either will resolve spontaneously or are easily treated by the primary care physician. Occasionally, the condition causing a red eye is a more serious disorder, such as intraocular inflammation, corneal inflammation, or acute glaucoma. A patient with one of these vision-threatening conditions requires the immediate attention of an ophthalmologist, because specialized skills, knowledge, and examining instruments are needed in order to make correct therapeutic decisions.

Basic Information

Red eye refers to hyperemia of the superficially visible vessels of the conjunctiva, episclera, and sclera. Hyperemia can be caused by disorders of these structures or of adjoining structures, including the cornea, the iris and ciliary body, and the adnexa. Specific disorders are discussed in the following section.

When to Examine

Any patient who complains of a red or painful eye should be examined to diagnose his condition as one of the following:

- acute angle-closure glaucoma **(Fig. 22):** rare form of glaucoma due to sudden and complete occlusion of the anterior chamber angle by iris tissue; serious. Note that the more common chronic open-angle glaucoma causes no redness of the eye. *(See Chapter 3, Chronic Visual Loss for discussion of glaucoma.)*

- iritis or iridocyclitis: inflammation of the iris alone or of the iris and ciliary body; often manifested by ciliary flush **(Fig. 23);** serious.

- herpes simplex keratitis **(Fig. 24):** inflammation of the cornea caused by herpes simplex virus; common, potentially serious; can lead to corneal ulceration.

- conjunctivitis **(Fig. 25):** hyperemia of the conjunctival blood vessels; may be bacterial, viral, allergic, or irritative; common, often not serious.

- episcleritis: inflammation of the episclera; less common, not serious, possibly allergic.

- scleritis **(Fig. 26):** inflammation of the sclera; less common, often protracted; may indicate serious systemic ocular disease such as collagen-vascular disorder; potentially serious to the eye.

- adnexal disease: affects the eyelids, lacrimal apparatus, and/or other appendages of the eye; includes dacryocystitis **(Fig. 27),** stye, and blepharitis. Red eye can also occur secondary to lid lesions, such as basal cell carcinoma or squamous cell carcinoma.

- other disorders, such as:
  - subconjunctival hemorrhage *(see Chapter 5, Injuries, Fig. 49).*
  - pterygium **(Fig. 28):** abnormal growth consisting of a triangular fold of tissue that advances progressively over the cornea, usually from the nasal side. Localized conjunctival inflammation may be associated with pterygium. Most cases occur in tropical climates. (Surgical excision is indicated if the pterygium starts to encroach on the visual axis.)

- ○ keratoconjunctivitis sicca: inflammation of the conjunctiva at the border of the cornea resulting from lacrimal deficiency; commonly called "dry eyes."
- ○ abrasions and foreign bodies: hyperemia can occur in response to corneal abrasions or foreign body injury.
- ○ secondary to abnormal lid function: Bell's palsy or other ocular exposure, such as that which occurs in some comatose patients, can result in a red eye.

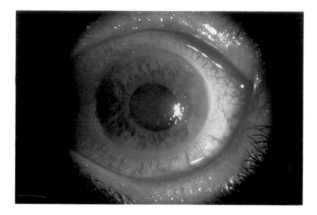

Fig. 22. Acute angle-closure glaucoma. The irregular corneal reflection and hazy appearance of the cornea suggest edema. However, the pupil is mid-dilated and the iris appears to be displaced anteriorly, with shallowing of the anterior chamber. Collectively, these findings plus an elevated intraocular pressure are diagnostic of acute angle-closure glaucoma.

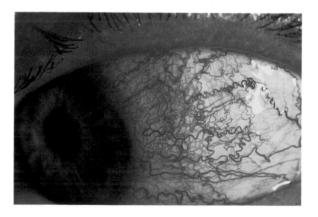

Fig. 23. Ciliary flush. Dilated deep conjunctival and episcleral vessels adjacent and circumferential to the corneal limbus cast a violet hue characteristic of ciliary flush and best seen in natural light.

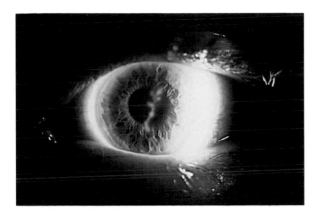

Fig. 24. Herpes simplex keratitis. In the center of the cornea is an irregular dendritic lesion of the corneal epithelium which is pathognomonic of herpes simplex.

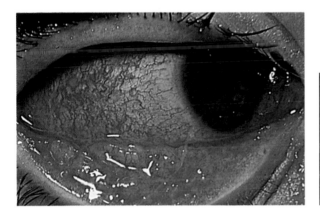

Fig. 25. Conjunctivitis. The hyperemia seen here is produced by a diffuse dilation of the conjunctival blood vessels. The dilation tends to be less intense in the perilimbal region. This is in contrast to the perilimbal dilation of deeper vessels characteristic of ciliary flush.

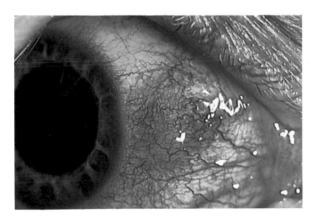

Fig. 26. Scleritis. This localized, raised, hyperemic lesion is characteristic of scleritis, which is associated with collagen, vascular, and rheumatoid diseases. Episcleritis appears flat, involves more superficial tissue, and is usually not associated with serious systemic disease. The etiology of episcleritis may be allergic.

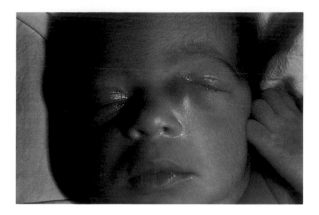

Fig. 27. Dacryocystitis. This obvious, raised, erythematous mass represents an acute inflammation of the lacrimal sac, usually secondary to a nasolacrimal duct obstruction. A purulent discharge may be extruded from the lid puncta by massage over the lacrimal sac.

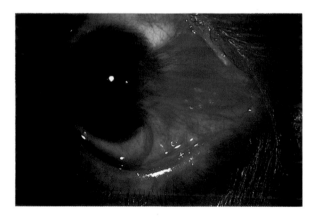

Fig. 28. Pterygium. This wedge-shaped growth of vascularized conjunctiva extends onto the cornea. The initial sign of pterygium may be a localized chronic conjunctivitis.

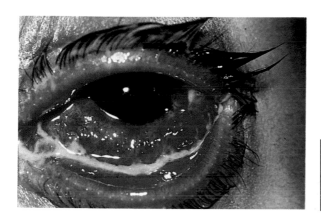

Fig. 29. Purulent conjunctivitis. With the lower lid everted, a creamy white exudate is visible, highlighted by the conjunctival hyperemia.

How to Examine *Know*

There are nine basic diagnostic techniques that must be mastered in order to evaluate a patient with a red eye.

- *Step 1.* Determine whether the visual acuity is normal or decreased, using a Snellen chart *(see Chapter 1, The Eye Examination).*

- *Step 2.* Decide by inspection whether the redness is due to subconjunctival hemorrhage, conjunctival hyperemia, ciliary flush, or a combination of these.

- *Step 3.* Detect the presence of conjunctival discharge and categorize it as to amount: profuse or scant; and character: purulent **(Fig. 29)**, mucopurulent, or serous.

- *Step 4.* Detect opacities of the cornea, including large keratic precipitates **(Fig. 30)** and/or irregularities of the corneal surface such as corneal edema, corneal leukoma, and irregular corneal reflection **(Figs. 31–33)**. Examination is done using a penlight or transilluminator.

- *Step 5.* Search for disruption of the corneal epithelium by staining the cornea with fluorescein.

- *Step 6.* Estimate the depth of the anterior chamber as normal or shallow; detect any blood or pus in the anterior chamber, which would indicate either hyphema or hypopyon, respectively. (Compare **Fig. 34,** *corneal ulcer with hypopyon, with the hyphema shown in Fig. 42 of Chapter 5, Injuries.)*

- *Step 7.* Detect irregularity of the pupils and determine if one pupil is larger or smaller than the other. Observe the reactivity of the pupils to light and to accommodation to determine whether one pupil is more sluggish than its mate or is nonreactive.

- *Step 8.* Determine whether the intraocular pressure is high, normal, or low using a Schiotz tonometer. (Tonometry is usually omitted when there is an obvious external infection.)

- *Step 9.* Detect the presence of proptosis **(Fig. 35)** and/or limitations of eye movement.

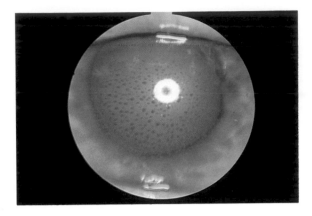

Fig. 30. Large keratic precipitates. Multiple gray-white opacities on the back surface of the cornea are seen against the background of the red reflex. These precipitates can result from chronic iridocyclitis.

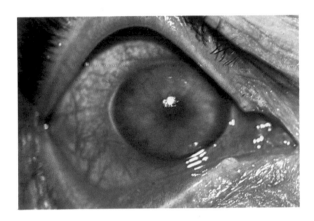

Fig. 31. Corneal edema. In this fiery red eye, the normally sharp corneal reflex is replaced by a diffuse, hazy appearance. Iris details are not as clear as usual.

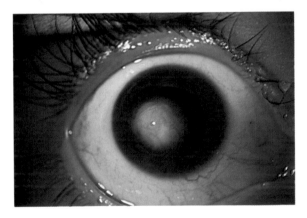

Fig. 32. Corneal leukoma. This dense, white corneal scar represents fibrosis secondary to a previous corneal insult, most frequently trauma or infection. If the scar encroaches on the visual axis, acuity may be impaired. Outside the scar the cornea is clear.

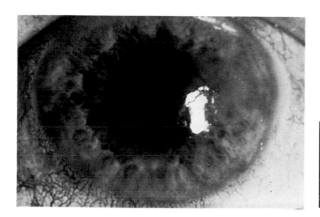

Fig. 33. Irregular corneal reflection. This localized irregularity of the normally sharp corneal light reflection indicates local disruption of the corneal epithelium.

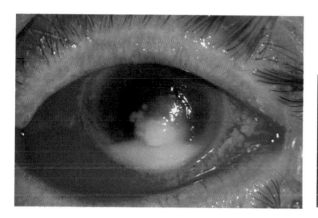

Fig. 34. Corneal ulcer with hypopyon. In this inflamed eye, one sees a white corneal opacity associated with an irregular corneal reflex. In addition, there is a prominent layering of white material in the inferior aspect of the anterior chamber, a hypopyon.

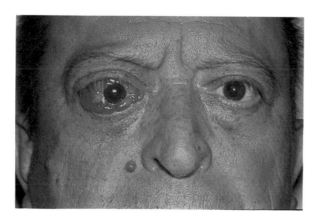

Fig. 35. Chronic proptosis. The right eye of this patient is proptotic, or anteriorly displaced. There is marked edema and hyperemia of the conjunctiva with tissue prolapse over the lower lid margin.

Interpreting the Findings

Although many conditions can cause a red eye and the associated signs and symptoms of the various disorders overlap to some extent, there are several signs and symptoms that signal danger. The presence of one or more of these danger signals should alert the physician that the patient has a disorder requiring an ophthalmologist's attention. **Tables 4.1** and **4.2** summarize significant signs and symptoms in the differential diagnosis of a red eye. In the discussion that follows, danger signals are marked with an asterisk (*).

Signs that Accompany a Red Eye

Ciliary flush. Ciliary flush **(see Fig. 23)** is an injection of the deep conjunctival and episcleral vessels surrounding the cornea. It is a danger sign often seen in eyes with corneal inflammations, iridocyclitis, or acute glaucoma. Usually, ciliary flush is not present in conjunctivitis. Ciliary flush is seen most easily in daylight and appears as a faint violet ring in which individual vessels are indiscernible to the unaided eye.

Conjunctival hyperemia. Conjunctival hyperemia **(see Fig. 25)** is an engorgement of the larger and more superficial bulbar conjunctival vessels. A nonspecific sign, it may be seen in almost any of the conditions causing a red eye.

Corneal opacification. In a patient with a red eye, corneal opacities always denote disease. These opacities may be detected by direct illumination with a penlight or they may be seen with a direct ophthalmoscope (with a plus lens in the viewing aperture) outlined against the red fundus reflex. Several types of corneal opacity may occur:

- A diffuse haze obscuring the pupil and iris markings, characteristic of corneal edema **(see Fig. 31)** and usually indicative of glaucoma;

- Localized opacities due to keratitis or ulcer **(see Fig. 32);**

- Keratic precipitates, or cellular deposits on the corneal endothelium, usually too small to be grossly visible but occasionally forming large clumps. These precipitates can result from iritis or from chronic iridocyclitis **(see Fig. 30).**

Corneal epithelial disruption. Disruption of the corneal epithelium occurs in corneal inflammations and trauma. It can be detected in two ways.

- *Method 1.* Position yourself so that you can observe the reflection from the cornea of a single light source (e.g., window, penlight) as the patient moves his eye into various positions. Epithelial disruptions cause distortion and irregularity of the reflection **(see Fig. 33).**

- *Method 2.* Apply fluorescein to the eye. Diseased epithelium or areas denuded of epithelium will stain a bright green. *(See Chapter 1, The Eye Examination, Fig. 5, and accompanying text for the technique of fluorescein staining.)*

Abnormalities of pupil size and shape. The pupil in an eye with iridocyclitis typically is somewhat smaller than that of the fellow eye due to reflex spasm of the iris sphincter muscle. The pupil is also distorted occasionally by posterior synechiae, which are inflammatory adhesions between the lens and iris. In acute glaucoma, the pupil is usually fixed, mid-dilated, and slightly irregular. Conjunctivitis, of course, does not affect the pupil.

Shallow anterior chamber. In a red eye , a shallow anterior chamber should always suggest the possibility of acute angle-closure glaucoma **(see Fig. 22).** Anterior chamber depth can be estimated through side illumination with a penlight. *(See Chapter 1, The Eye Examination, for details on estimating the depth of the anterior chamber.)*

Intraocular pressure. Intraocular pressure is unaffected by common causes of red eye other than iridocyclitis and glaucoma. In any red eye without obvious infection, the intraocular pressure should be measured to rule out glaucoma. *(See Chapter 1, The Eye Examination, for the use of Schiotz tonometry to measure intraocular pressure.)*

Proptosis. Proptosis is a forward displacement of the globe. Sudden proptosis suggests serious orbital or cavernous sinus disease. The most common cause of chronic proptosis **(see Fig. 35)** is thyroid disease; however, orbital mass lesions also result in proptosis and should be ruled out early in the diagnosis. Small amounts of proptosis are detected most easily by standing behind the seated patient and looking down to compare the positions of the two corneas.

Discharge. The type of discharge or exudate may be an important clue to the etiology of a patient's conjunctivitis. Purulent (creamy white, **see Fig. 29**) or mucopurulent (yellowish) exudate suggests a bacterial etiology. Serous (watery, clear or yellow-tinged) discharge suggests a viral etiology. Scant, white, stringy exudate sometimes occurs in allergic conjunctivitis and in keratoconjunctivitis sicca, a condition commonly known as "dry eyes."

Preauricular lymph node enlargement. Enlargement of the lymph nodes just in front of the auricle of the ear is a frequent sign of viral conjunctivitis. Usually, such enlargement does not occur in acute bacterial conjunctivitis. Preauricular node enlargement can be a prominent feature of some unusual varieties of chronic granulomatous conjunctivitis, known collectively as Parinaud's oculoglandular syndrome. The chief causes of this syndrome include chancre, tuberculosis, lymphogranuloma venereum, leptotrichosis, and tularemia.

Symptoms that Accompany a Red Eye

Blurred vision. Blurred vision that does not disappear on blinking suggests a serious ocular disease such as an inflamed cornea, iridocyclitis, or glaucoma. It never occurs in simple conjunctivitis unless there is associated corneal involvement.

Table 4.1. Signs of Red Eye

Signs	Referral advisable if abnormal	Acute glaucoma	Acute iridocyclitis	Keratitis	Bacterial conjunctivitis	Viral conjunctivitis	Allergic conjunctivitis
Ciliary flush	Yes	1	2	3	0	0	0
Conjunctival injection	No	2	2	2	3	2	1
Corneal opacification	Yes	3	0	1 to 3	0	0 or 1	0
Corneal epithelial disruption	Yes	0	0	1 to 3	0	0 or 1	0
Pupil	Yes	Mid-dilated, nonreactive	Small, may be irregular	Normal or small	Normal	Normal	Normal
Anterior chamber depth	Yes	Shallow	Normal	Normal	Normal	Normal	Normal
Intraocular pressure	Yes	High	Usually low	Normal	Normal	Normal	Normal
Proptosis	Yes	0	0	0	0	0	0
Discharge	No	0	0	Sometimes	2 or 3	2	1
Preauricular lymph node	No	0	0	0	0	1	0

Note: The range of severity is indicated by 0 (absent) to 3 (severe).

Table 4.2. Symptoms of Red Eye

Symptoms	Referral advisable if present	Acute glaucoma	Acute iridocyclitis	Keratitis	Bacterial conjunctivitis	Viral conjunctivitis	Allergic conjunctivitis
Blurred vision	Yes	3	1 to 2	3	0	0	0
Pain	Yes	2 to 3	2	2	0	0	0
Photophobia	Yes	1	3	3	0	0	0
Colored halos	Yes	2	0	0	0	0	0
Exudation	No	0	0	0 to 3	3	2	1
Itching	No	0	0	0	0	0	2

Note: The range of severity is indicated by 0 (absent) to 3 (severe).

Pain. Pain may indicate keratitis, ulcer, iridocyclitis, or acute glaucoma. Patients with conjunctivitis may complain of a scratchiness or mild irritation but not of severe pain.

Photophobia. Photophobia is an abnormal sensitivity to light that accompanies iritis, either alone or secondary to corneal inflammation. Patients with conjunctivitis have normal light sensitivity.

Colored halos. Rainbow-like fringes, or colored halos, seen around a point of light are usually a symptom of corneal edema, often resulting from an abrupt rise in intraocular pressure. Therefore, colored halos are a danger symptom suggesting acute glaucoma as the cause of a red eye.

Exudation. Exudation, also called mattering, is a typical result of conjunctival or eyelid inflammations and does not occur in iridocyclitis or glaucoma. Patients will often complain that their lids are "stuck together" on awakening from sleep. Corneal ulcer is a serious condition that may or may not be accompanied by exudate.

Itching. Although a nonspecific symptom, itching usually indicates allergic conjunctivitis.

Associated Systemic Problems

- *Upper respiratory infection and fever.* Infection of the upper respiratory tract accompanied by fever may be associated with conjunctivitis, particularly when these symptoms are due to adenovirus type 3 or type 7 (both of which cause pharyngoconjunctival fever). Allergic conjunctivitis may be associated with the seasonal rhinitis of hay fever.

- *Erythema multiforme.* Erythema multiforme is a serious systemic disorder, possibly an allergic response to medication, which can result in severe conjunctivitis, irreversible conjunctival scarring, and blindness. Stevens-Johnson syndrome is the name given to this form of erythema multiforme with ocular involvement.

Laboratory Diagnosis

In practice, most cases of conjunctivitis are managed without laboratory assistance. This represents a compromise with ideal management but is justified by the economic waste of obtaining routine smears and cultures in such a common and benign disease. Most clinicians, after making a presumptive clinical diagnosis of bacterial conjunctivitis, proceed directly to broad-spectrum topical ophthalmic antibiotic treatment. Cases of presumed bacterial conjunctivitis which do not improve in two days with antibiotic treatment should be referred to an ophthalmologist for confirmation of the diagnosis and appropriate laboratory studies.

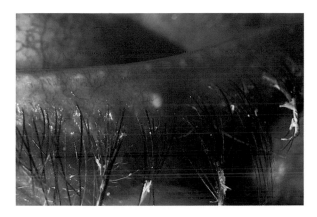

Fig. 36. Staphylococcal blepharitis. Chronic staphylococcal lid infection produces inflamed, swollen lids which may ulcerate. The oily discharge binds the lashes and sometimes condenses to form a collarette around a lash.

Smears and scrapings. In doubtful cases, smears of exudate or conjunctival scrapings can confirm clinical impressions regarding the type of conjunctivitis. Typical findings include polymorphonuclear cells and bacteria in bacterial conjunctivitis, lymphocytes in viral conjunctivitis, and eosinophils in allergic conjunctivitis.

Cultures. Cultures for bacteria and determinations of antibiotic sensitivity are also useful in cases resistant to therapy.

Management or Referral

The following conditions either require no treatment or may be appropriately treated by a primary care physician. Of course, cases requiring prolonged treatment or those in which the expected response to treatment does not occur promptly should be referred to an ophthalmologist.

Blepharitis. Response to the treatment of blepharitis is often frustratingly slow, and relapses are common. The mainstays of treatment are

- eradication of staphylococcal infection **(Fig. 36)** with frequent applications of appropriate antibiotic eyedrops or ointment.
- treatment of scalp seborrhea with antidandruff shampoos to prevent the spread of seborrhea to the eyes;
- cleansing of the lids to alleviate seborrheic blepharitis **(Fig. 37).**

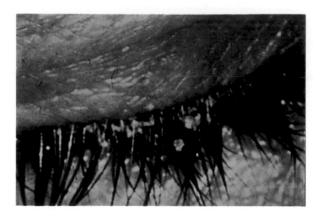

Fig. 37. Seborrheic blepharitis. The dry, flaky lashes and red lid margins seen here are characteristic of seborrheic blepharitis.

Stye. A stye, or hordeolum, is an acute infection of the eyelid which may be characterized as external (involving the hair follicle or associated glands of Zeis or Moll) or as internal (involving the meibomian glands). An external hordeolum **(Fig. 38)** occurs on the surface of the skin at the edge of the lid. An internal hordeolum **(Fig. 39)** presents on the conjunctival surface of the lid. A chalazion **(Fig. 40)** is a chronic granulomatous inflammation of a meibomian gland which may develop spontaneously or may follow an internal hordeolum.

Treatment consists of frequently applied warm compresses, and incision and drainage when the stye comes to a point. Sulfonamides or other antibiotics are often applied locally to treat associated blepharitis and to lessen the chance that other sebaceous glands will become infected. Persistent or recurring lid masses should be biopsied since they represent the rare meibomian gland carcinoma or squamous carcinoma of the conjunctiva, rather than a benign chalazion **(see Fig. 40).**

Subconjunctival hemorrhage. In the absence of blunt trauma, hemorrhage into the subconjunctiva requires no treatment and, unless recurrent, no evaluation. *(For figure of subconjunctival hemorrhage, see Chapter 5, Injuries, Fig. 49.)*

Conjunctivitis. Bacterial conjunctivitis is treated with frequent antibiotic eyedrops as well as antibiotic ointment applied before bedtime. Cool compresses may give some relief. There is no specific treatment for viral conjunctivitis. It cannot be emphasized too strongly, however, that corticosteroids have no place in the treatment of infectious conjunctivitis and that eyedrops containing a combination of antibiotics and corticosteroids are seldom if ever indicated for the treatment of any ocular inflammation.

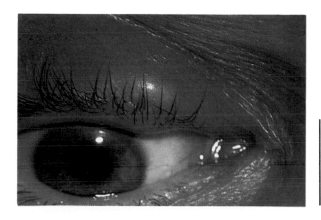

Fig. 38. External hordeolum. This large, acute swelling, which is red and painful, involves the hair follicles or associated glands of Zeis or Moll, and points toward the skin.

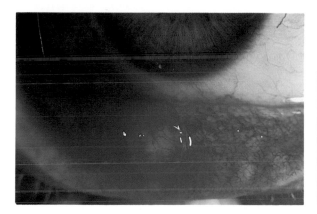

Fig. 39. Internal hordeolum. An acute infection of a meibomian gland produces a swelling directed internally toward the conjunctiva. This figure demonstrates a discrete circumscribed area of inflammation highlighted by a hyperemic conjunctiva.

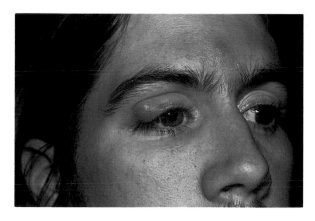

Fig. 40. Chalazion. This large, nontender lid mass is a chronic granulomatous inflammation of a meibomian gland.

Therapeutic Warnings

Topical Anesthetics

Topical anesthetics should never be prescribed for prolonged analgesia in ocular inflammations and injuries for three reasons:

- Topical anesthetics inhibit growth and healing of the corneal epithelium.
- Topical anesthetics may cause severe allergic reactions.
- Corneal anesthesia eliminates the protective blink reflex, exposing the cornea to dehydration and injury.

Topical Corticosteroids

Topical corticosteroids have three potentially serious ocular side effects.

- *Keratitis.* Herpes simplex keratitis **(see Fig. 24)** and fungal keratitis are both markedly potentiated by corticosteroids. Corticosteroids may mask symptoms of inflammation, making the patient "feel" better, while the cornea may be melting away or even perforating.
- *Cataracts.* Prolonged use of corticosteroids, either locally or systemically, will often lead to cataract formation.
- *Elevated intraocular pressure.* Local application of corticosteroids for two to six weeks may cause an elevation of intraocular pressure in approximately one third of the population. The pressure rise may be severe in a small percentage of cases. Optic nerve damage and loss of vision can occur.

The combination of a corticosteroid and an antibiotic carries the same risk. Topical corticosteroids alone, or in combination with other antibiotics, should not be administered to the eye by a primary care physician. They can be very helpful when used under the close supervision of an ophthalmologist.

Sample Problems

1. A twenty-three-year-old school teacher complains that her right eye is red and irritated. You note moderate injection of the larger conjunctival vessels, watery discharge, and a palpable preauricular lymph node.

   Question a: From this information alone, what tentative diagnosis would you make?

Answer: The conjunctival injection and discharge suggest conjunctivitis. The serous nature of the discharge plus the preauricular adenopathy indicate that she has viral conjunctivitis.

Question b: Again based on the above information, which of the following symptoms might be elicited by a careful history?

(1) blurred vision
(2) sore throat
(3) history of exposure to school children with colds
(4) itching

Answer: Sore throat often accompanies viral conjunctivitis; in such cases, a history of exposure to other individuals with upper respiratory infections can often be elicited. Blurred vision, a danger signal, is not a feature of conjunctivitis. Itching is a symptom of allergic, not viral, conjunctivitis.

Question c: Which of the following are also possible findings in this case?

(1) a smaller pupil in the right eye
(2) lymphocytes in a smear of conjunctival scrapings
(3) keratic precipitates

Answer: A small pupil and keratic precipitates are signs of iritis. Lymphocytes are usually found in scrapings from eyes with viral conjunctivitis.

Question d: Management by a primary care physician should consist of which of the following?

(1) corticosteroid drops
(2) broad spectrum antibiotic drops
(3) referral to an ophthalmologist
(4) instruction to the patient to stay home from school until the redness resolves

Answer: There is no specific treatment for viral conjunctivitis. Corticosteroids are contraindicated. Because the disease is contagious, the patient should be instructed to remain home from work.

2. A man returned recently from an African journey. During his trip he had three episodes of blurring and pain in his left eye that each lasted about two hours and were relieved by sleep. A few hours before seeing you, his symptoms recurred.

Question a: Which of the following signs convince you that the patient does not have some bizarre variety of tropical conjunctivitis?

(1) visual acuity of 20/200 in the left eye
(2) conjunctival injection
(3) ciliary flush
(4) absence of exudate

Answer: Blurred vision and ciliary flush are danger signals of serious ocular disease. The absence of exudate is also evidence against conjunctivitis.

Question b: You note a diffuse haziness of the patient's left cornea. What is the most likely diagnosis?

Answer: Diffuse haziness of the cornea is usually due to edema. This and the history of recurrent attacks relieved by sleep suggest the diagnosis of acute angle-closure glaucoma.

Question c: You seek confirmatory data for your tentative diagnosis. What would you expect the following tests to show if your diagnosis were correct?

(1) estimation of anterior chamber depth: deep or shallow?
(2) pupil diameter: large or small?
(3) intraocular pressure: high or low?

Answer: In angle-closure glaucoma, the anterior chamber is shallow, the pupil is usually mid-dilated, and the intraocular pressure is high.

Question d: Your management should be which of the following?

(1) corticosteroid eyedrops
(2) advice to see an ophthalmologist the next day
(3) a telephone request to an ophthalmologist for immediate examination

Answer: Angle-closure glaucoma requires emergency treatment to lower the intraocular pressure. The patient should be referred immediately to an ophthalmologist. If an ophthalmologist is not immediately available, you may begin topical pilocarpine hydrochloride 1% or 2% (*Isopto® Carpine*); a topical beta-adrenergic blocker; and a systemic carbonic anhydrase inhibitor. *(See Chapter 9, Drugs and the Eye, for details on these drugs.)*

3. After working in his garden, a fifty-seven-year-old man complains of moderate discomfort and redness in his right eye. You note a visual acuity of 20/25 in the right eye, and of 20/15 in the left eye. The right eye has mild hyperemia of the conjunctival vessels; the right cornea appears clear to penlight examination.

   It is not one of your better days. You diagnose a probable allergy to pollen and advise the patient to use dexamethasone sodium phosphate 0.1% (*Decadron®*) for three days.

Question a: Give two reasons why your diagnosis of allergic conjunctivitis is unlikely to be correct.

Answer: Unless the patient has always had weaker vision in his right eye, this finding should alert you to the possibility of a more serious inflammation such as iridocyclitis, keratitis, or glaucoma. Also, the patient does not complain of itching, which you might expect in an allergic reaction.

Question b: What other diagnostic techniques should you have performed to be certain that the cornea is normal?

Answer: If the patient has an early herpes simplex keratitis or if his cornea has been scratched by a twig, the epithelial disruption might not be easily seen during a quick penlight examination. However, it most likely would be rendered visible by fluorescein staining of the cornea.

Question c: Is there any hazard in your prescribed course of treatment?

Answer: The virulence of both herpes simplex and fungal infections, which can result from trauma involving organic material, is markedly potentiated by the application of topical corticosteroids to the eye.

Annotated References

1. Duane TD, Jaeger EA (eds): *Clinical Ophthalmology.* Philadelphia, Harper & Row, 1985, vol 4.

   Updated, comprehensive discussion of external disease and uveitis.

2. Duke-Elder S (ed): Diseases of the outer eye: Part I: Conjunctiva; Part II: Cornea and sclera, in *System of Ophthalmology.* St. Louis, Mo, CV Mosby Co, 1965, vol 8, parts 1 & 2.

   An extremely comprehensive discussion of external disease with historical perspective and anecdotes.

3. Peyman GA, Sanders DR, Goldberg MF (eds): *Principles and Practice of Ophthalmology.* Philadelphia, WB Saunders Co, 1980, vol 1.

   Chapter 5 (Infections of the Ocular Adnexa) provides a good, detailed discussion of various infectious agents and their particular manifestations.

4. Scheie HG, Albert DM: *Textbook of Ophthalmology,* ed 9. Philadelphia, WB Saunders Co, 1977.

   Chapter 14 (Medical Ophthalmology) provides a basic discussion of external disease.

5. Vaughan D, Asbury T: *General Ophthalmology,* ed 11. Los Altos, Calif, Lange Medical Publications, 1986.

   Covers differential diagnosis of red eye and external disease.

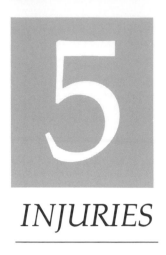

INJURIES

Objective

The primary care physician should be able to evaluate the common ocular or orbital injuries and determine whether or not the problem requires the prompt attention of an ophthalmologist. Even in situations of true ocular emergency, such as chemical burns, you should be able to institute therapy where appropriate.

To achieve this objective you should learn:

- To recognize which problems are urgent. Do not waste time obtaining a prolonged history if urgent treatment is indicated. Chemical burns of the eye, penetrating injuries of the globe, lid lacerations, and hyphemas are urgent.

- Which salient facts to obtain. These include the time of injury; the place of injury; the circumstances of occurrence (e.g., blunt or sharp trauma, acid or alkali burn); and the history of eye conditions, drug allergies, and tetanus immunization.

- How to examine the traumatized eye and record the visual acuity as accurately as possible.

- Whether to manage or to refer the most common injuries likely to be seen by a primary care physician.

Relevance

One day, whether in your own home or yard or while on duty in the emergency center, you will be confronted with an unexpected ocular injury. The purpose of this chapter is to assist you in developing confidence when approaching minor or major eye injuries; it will further your competence in acquiring the basic techniques and knowledge necessary to assess and initiate treatment of the eye and its surrounding structures.

Basic Information

To deal effectively with eye injuries, you must be familiar with the anatomy and function of the eye and its surrounding structures.

- Bony orbit
  - ○ The margins of the orbit protect the globe from impact with large objects.
  - ○ A marginal fracture usually causes no decrease in function.
  - ○ The very thin orbital floor may "blow out" into the maxillary sinus from blunt impact to the orbit, from a fist or tennis ball, for instance. Orbital contents, including the inferior rectus and inferior oblique muscles, may become trapped, restricting vertical eye movement and causing double vision (i.e., diplopia).
  - ○ A medial fracture of the thin ethmoidal bone may be associated with subcutaneous emphysema of the eyelids.
  - ○ A fracture at or near the optic canal, through which the optic nerve and ophthalmic artery pass, may cause damage to the optic nerve, with resulting visual loss.
- Lids
  - ○ The lids close reflexively when the eyes are threatened.
  - ○ The act of blinking keeps the cornea clear, through constant surface contact and tear production.
  - ○ In the case of a facial nerve palsy, the globe may be exposed to drying or other injury.
  - ○ Lid margins must be intact to ensure proper lid closure and tear drainage.
- Lacrimal apparatus. Tear drainage occurs at the medial aspect of the lids, primarily through the lower lacrimal punctum, and continues through the canaliculi to the lacrimal sac, and via the nasolacrimal duct to the nose *(see Chapter 1, The Eye Examination, Illus. 1.2)*. Failure to recognize and properly repair a lower canalicular laceration can result in chronic tearing (i.e., epiphora).
- Conjunctiva and cornea
  - ○ The corneal epithelium usually heals quickly following abrasion.
  - ○ Small lacerations of the conjunctiva heal quickly and, consequently, may conceal a penetrating injury of the globe.
- Anterior chamber. The aqueous humor often escapes in penetrating injuries; this can result in a "shallow" or "flat" chamber.
- Iris and ciliary body
  - ○ Following laceration of the cornea or limbus, the iris may prolapse into the wound **(Fig. 41),** resulting in an irregular pupil.

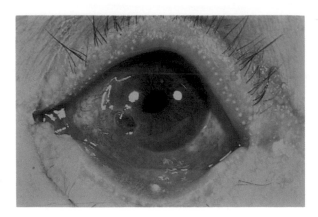

Fig. 41. Corneal perforation with iris prolapse. Slight distortion of the pupil, irregularity of the corneal reflection, and a knuckle of soft, brown tissue at the limbus indicate a corneal perforation through which the iris has prolapsed.

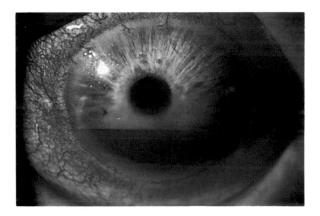

Fig. 42. Hyphema. In the anterior chamber at the six o'clock position a dark pool of blood with a flat top is visible. Note also the conjunctival hyperemia.

- ○ Blunt trauma to the eyeball may produce iritis, resulting in pain, redness, photophobia, and a small pupil (i.e., miosis).
- ○ Contusions may deform the pupil by tearing the iris root or by notching the pupillary margin.
- ○ Contusions may result in tearing of small vessels in the anterior chamber angle, causing hemorrhage into the anterior chamber (i.e., hyphema, **Fig. 42**). A hyphema is generally the result of trauma and usually resolves spontaneously.

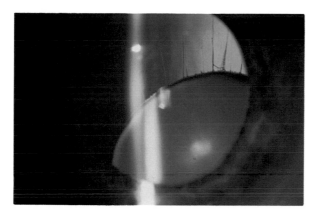

Fig. 43. Subluxated lens. Light reflected off the fundus and back through a dilated pupil silhouettes the edge of a subluxated lens with stretched zonular fibers. Ordinarily, the edge of the lens is not visible even if the pupil is widely dilated.

- Lens
  - Injuries to the lens proceed most often to cataract formation.
  - Blunt trauma to the globe can cause a partial dislocation (i.e., subluxation) of the lens **(Fig. 43).**
- Vitreous humor. Loss of transparency may result from hemorrhage and infection.
- Retina
  - The retina is protected exteriorly by the sclera, a tough outer layer, and the choroid, an underlying vascular layer.
  - The retina is thin and vulnerable. If the surface is scratched or penetrated by a foreign body, retinal detachment from the pigment epithelium may occur *(see Chapter 2, Acute Visual Loss, Fig. 6).*
  - Retinal hemorrhage may develop as a result of direct or indirect trauma.
  - The retina turns white when edematous.
  - Macular damage will reduce visual acuity without producing complete blindness.

When to Examine

Most ocular injuries present with obvious redness and pain. However, some injuries provide few warning signs. For example, a sharp perforation may produce minimal redness and escape attention. The examiner should be especially alert to perforating injuries caused by small pieces of metal chipped off when metal hits metal. A foreign body **(Fig. 44)** in the posterior segment produces no pain since the lens, retina, and vitreous have no nerve endings to conduct sensations of pain, although all other structures of the eyeball do.

If disease of the posterior segment is suspected, including retinal detachment and/or intraocular foreign body, referral to an ophthalmologist is indicated. It will facilitate the ophthalmologist's examination of the fundus if you do not use ointment in the eye.

How to Examine/Interpreting the Findings

For an eye injury, you should perform and record a complete examination of the eyes and surrounding structures, to include visual acuity, external examination, the pupils, eye movements, and ophthalmoscopy.

Visual Acuity

You must record visual acuity as specifically as possible. Refer to *Chapter 1, The Eye Examination,* for instructions on the use of the Snellen eye chart. If a Snellen chart is unavailable, determine the patient's ability to read available print material and record the type of print used (e.g., newspaper, telephone book) and the distance at which it was read. Note in particular if vision is equal in both eyes. If vision is below reading level, determine the patient's ability to count fingers, perceive hand motions, and respond to light; note also the direct and consensual pupillary reactions.

External Examination

An examination of the external structures of the eye should include:

Palpation. Palpation of the orbital rim(s) should be performed if a question of blunt injury or fracture exists.

Penlight inspection. A penlight is used to inspect the eye for signs of perforation, such as reduced depth of the anterior chamber or uveal prolapse **(see Fig. 41).** Hyphema **(see Fig. 42)** may be present without perforation and, in fact, often accompanies blunt injury.

Lid eversion. Retraction and eversion of the upper and lower eyelids will facilitate inspection for a foreign body or chemical burn. Do not manipulate the eyelids if you suspect a penetrating injury of the globe.

Fluorescein staining. If the patient has foreign body sensation, or if there is a history of blunt or sharp injury, fluorescein is used to stain the cornea to identify any corneal epithelial defects. *(See Chapter 1, The Eye Examination, for the technique of fluorescein staining.)*

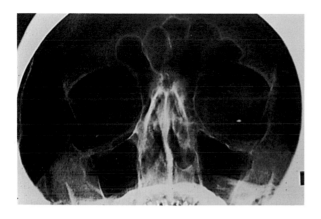

Fig. 44. Roentgenogram of foreign body. In the left orbit, a small radiopaque foreign body is visible.

Anesthesia. Drops can be used to provide topical anesthesia, especially to relieve foreign body sensation or discomfort, due to prolonged wear of contact lenses or sunburn, for example. Use of one drop of proparacaine hydrochloride 0.5% *(Ophthaine®)* will provide almost instantaneous pain relief and allow you to proceed with an adequate evaluation, including determination of visual acuity, which would be otherwise impossible due to discomfort. Do not prescribe anesthetic drops or ointment because prolonged use can result in corneal ulceration and inadvertent injury *(see Chapter 9, Drugs and the Eye).*

Pupils

Always check for afferent pupillary defect in trauma cases. Diminished direct pupillary reaction to light with an intact consensual response may indicate an optic nerve injury *(see Chapter 7, Neuro-Ophthalmology).*

Eye Movements

Movement of the eye may be generally restricted in the case of orbital hematoma. Vertical restriction combined with vertical diplopia should make you suspect a blowout fracture. If limitation of eye movements is accompanied by proptosis, auscultate the head and eye for a bruit, which would be suggestive of carotid-cavernous sinus fistula.

Ophthalmoscopy

Conditions that indicate referral. If the fundus is visible, look for edema, retinal hemorrhages, retinal detachment, and, if penetration is suspected, a foreign body. In the event of a positive finding or the suspicion of a penetrating injury or foreign body, refer the patient to an ophthalmologist immediately.

No red reflex. The normal red reflex from the fundus is evenly colored and not interrupted by shadows *(see Chapter 1, The Eye Examination, Fig. 1).* If the red reflex is absent, immediate referral to an ophthalmologist is dictated. Usually, absence of the red reflex is due to one of the following conditions: (1) hyphema in the anterior chamber, (2) cataract from acute swelling of the lens, or (3) vitreous hemorrhage.

Hyphema and cataract are visible on external examination with a penlight, whereas the detection of vitreous hemorrhage requires fundus examination and assessment of the red reflex with a direct ophthalmoscope.

X Rays

Radiological evaluation is suggested if there is any question of facial or orbital fracture or of possible ocular or orbital foreign body.

Sample Examinations

In the evaluation of ocular injuries, it is important to document the time and nature of the event as well as the onset of symptomatology. After significant trauma has occurred, the person may be unconscious or unable to answer questions. As in any trauma situation, you should not delay prompt treatment for a prolonged history if an obvious injury, such as a chemical burn, exists. Two sample examinations are provided in **Tables 5.1** and **5.2.**

Management or Referral

The primary care physician may not be able to provide definitive care for each of the entities discussed below, but should be able to initiate treatment in every case.

True emergencies. Therapy must be instituted within minutes. Chemical burns of the conjunctiva and cornea represent one of the true ocular emergencies. An alkali burn **(Fig. 45)** usually results in greater damage to the eye than an acid burn, since alkali compounds (e.g., lye, anhydrous ammonia) penetrate ocular tissues more rapidly. All chemical burns require immediate and profuse irrigation, followed by referral to an ophthalmologist.

Urgent situation. Therapy should be instituted within a few hours. Any of the following conditions constitutes an urgent situation.

- Penetrating injuries of the globe, whether actual or suspected, necessitate the protection of an eye shield. Neither a patch nor ointment is required. X rays of the orbit to check for radiopaque foreign bodies **(see Fig. 44)** should be ordered. Referral to an ophthalmologist is indicated.

- For conjunctival or corneal foreign bodies **(Figs. 46, 47),** anesthetize with proparacaine 0.5% and try to remove any loose foreign bodies with a cotton-tipped applicator. Refer patients with any residual embedded foreign bodies to an ophthalmologist.

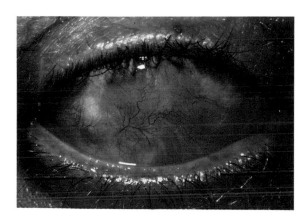

Fig. 45. Severe alkali burn. Damage includes total opacification of the cornea, with growth of superficial vessels from the conjunctiva into the corneal scar, and surrounding bulbar hyperemia.

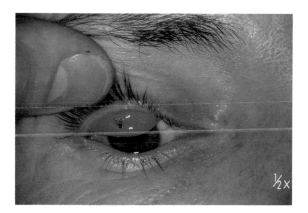

Fig. 46. Conjunctival foreign body. Foreign bodies often lodge under the edge of the upper eyelid. As this figure shows, they are easily seen and removed upon eversion of the eyelid.

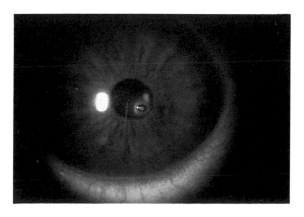

Fig. 47. Corneal foreign body. Visible here is a small piece of rusty iron embedded in the surface of the cornea. Surrounding the iron is a ring of grayish corneal edema.

Table 5.1. Sample Examination: Foreign Body Sensation

History

Type of injury, time, and place	3:15 a.m., seen in emergency center.
Appropriate chain of events. Is trauma centered in the right eye (OD), in the left eye (OS), or is it bilateral (OU)?	At approximately 2:45 a.m., patient awoke with severe foreign body sensation OU.
Subjective visual loss, if any, and amount of visual decrease. Was vision normal prior to injury? *Associated complaints* *Symptoms*	No injury, although admits to using sun lamp to tan face for twenty minutes previous evening. Now unable to open eyes which aggravates burning foreign body sensation. Unable to see well but uncertain about degree of visual loss.

Examination

Best correctable visual acuity (VA) for both eyes, i.e., with glasses if available, with pinhole if necessary	Unable to cooperate until 1 drop proparacaine 0.5% administered OU. VA: OD 20/25; OS 20/20.
Appearance and function of: *Lids and bony orbit*	Bony orbit intact but marked eyelid spasm until anesthetic drops given.
Cornea and conjunctiva	Cornea stains irregularly with fluorescein. Conjunctival injection OU; pronounced near limbus.
Media (aqueous, lens, vitreous)	Media clear on gross inspection.

Diagnosis

	Ultraviolet conjunctival and corneal injury.

Management

	Homatropine hydrobromide 2% (Homatrocel®) drops, antibiotic ointment, and moderate pressure dressing.

Table 5.2. Sample Examination: Double Vision

History

The approximate onset of symptoms	A sixteen-year-old boy complains that he awoke two days ago with fullness in the left eye. Later, he noted vertical double vision when looking straight up, up and right, and up and left; no double vision when looking straight ahead. No other problem except mild aching when looking up. Hit by knee in left eye in wrestling class three days prior.
Type of symptoms, frequency, regularity	
Increasing or decreasing severity?	

Examination

Ocular findings	Perform complete eye examination, with particular attention to testing extraocular muscles. Rule out possible damage to globe.
X rays	Obtain Waters view and, if necessary, tomograms of the orbits in the Waters position to look for opacification of the maxillary antrum and downward herniation of orbital structures.

Diagnosis

	Blowout fracture left orbit with muscle entrapment.

Management

	Call ophthalmologist.

- For corneal abrasions, take the following steps:

  (1) anesthetize with proparacaine 0.5%;

  (2) perform gross examination;

  (3) stain with fluorescein to enhance view;

  (4) instill antibiotic drops; instill short-acting cycloplegic drops for the relief of pain as indicated;

  (5) patch; and

  (6) recheck in twenty-four hours.

  Refer severe cases to an ophthalmologist. *(For figure of fluorescein stain delineating corneal abrasion, see Chapter 1, The Eye Examination, Fig. 5.)*

- Hyphema requires referral to an ophthalmologist. *(See Chapter 2, Acute Visual Loss, for further discussion.)*

- A lid laceration can be sutured if not deep, and if there is no involvement of the lid margin or canaliculi; otherwise, refer to an ophthalmologist. (The lid laceration shown in **Fig. 48** requires referral since it is full thickness and involves the lid margin. There is also a possibility of canalicular involvement because the laceration is close to the medial canthus.)

- Radiant energy burns, such as welder's burn or snow blindness, require anesthesia, examination, antibiotics, and a patch.

Semiurgent condition. Refer to an ophthalmologist within one to two days. An orbital fracture falls into this category.

Nonurgent condition. No referral is necessary. Subconjunctival hemorrhage **(Fig. 49)** in the absence of blunt trauma is a nonurgent condition. These hemorrhages are resorbed spontaneously and require no evaluation unless they are recurrent.

Treatment Skills

The following are the treatment skills that every physician needs in order to properly manage eye injuries.

- Ocular irrigation. Plastic squeeze bottles **(Fig. 50)** of eye irrigation solutions, or normal saline IV drip with plastic tubing, are ideal for ocular irrigation. Irrigation may be facilitated by the use of a topical anesthetic. However, first aid for chemical injuries of the eye may demand the earliest possible irrigation using any source of water available, such as a garden hose, drinking fountain, or faucet. It cannot be overstated that chemical burns require immediate and profuse irrigation.

- Foreign bodies. Removal of a foreign body from the cornea or conjunctiva is done with a cotton-tipped applicator, following application of an anesthetic, such as proparacaine 0.5%.

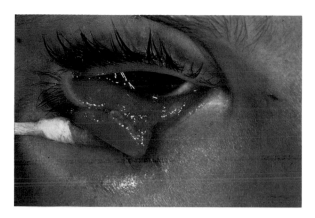

Fig. 48. Full thickness lid laceration. The lower eyelid is partially everted with the applicator stick, revealing an irregular laceration of the lid margin, orbicularis muscle, tarsal plate, and conjunctiva. Note the proximity of the laceration to the medial canthus, indicating possible canalicular involvement.

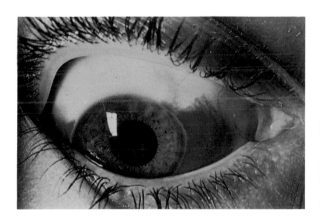

Fig. 49. Subconjunctival hemorrhage. This circumscribed hemorrhage is located between the conjunctiva and sclera; its bright red color and sudden appearance are characteristic.

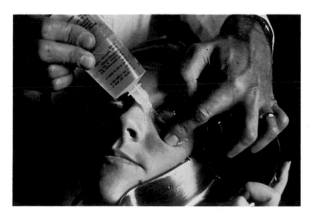

Fig. 50. Irrigation. Here, the examiner uses a plastic squeeze bottle of water or normal saline to irrigate the eye. The patient is instructed to look in various directions while the opposite portions of the conjunctival cul-de-sac are flushed vigorously.

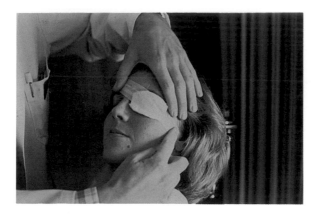

Fig. 51. Patch. The patient is instructed to close her eye while one or more oval, gauze eye patches are taped firmly enough to immobilize the lid in a closed position. Note the oblique placement of the tape so that jaw movement is unlikely to loosen it.

- Eye medications
  - Cycloplegics. Homatropine 2% or cyclopentolate hydrochloride 1% (*Cyclogyl®*) may be used to relax the iris and ciliary body and to relieve the pain and discomfort of most forms of nonpenetrating ocular injuries. Longer-acting cycloplegics, atropine for example, are usually not needed. *(See Chapter 9, Drugs and the Eye, for further discussion of cycloplegics.)*
  - Antibiotic ointment. In general, if employed for one-time use in clean wounds, antibiotic ointments can be used without side-effects. If more frequent use is necessary, one must be concerned about allergic reactions and/or superinfections.
  - Anesthetic drops and ointment. Ocular anesthetics should never be prescribed for home use because of the tendency for overuse by the patient.
  - Corticosteroid drops and ointment. Corticosteroids should not be administered for ocular injuries by the primary care physician since there is a major risk of severe corneal damage with continued use *(see Chapter 9, Drugs and the Eye)*.
- Patching
  - Light patch. A light patch often makes a patient more comfortable following minor eye injuries. This type of patch consists of a single sterile eye pad applied with several strips of tape **(Fig. 51)**.
  - Pressure patch. A moderate pressure patch is utilized following injuries that affect the corneal epithelium, for example corneal abrasions, and after removal of foreign bodies. An eye patch plus a fluffed piece of gauze or two patches are applied by putting moderate tension on the strips of tape used. Make sure the patch is tight enough to prevent the patient from accidentally opening his eye under it; once the anesthesia has worn off, such friction would be extremely painful.

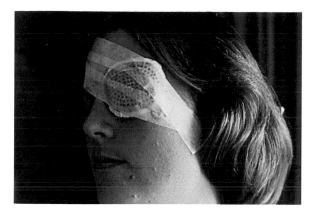

Fig. 52. Shield. Shown here is the Fox shield, made of malleable metal and perforated. The shield is carefully shaped so that it is supported by the rim of the orbit when taped in place.

- ○ Shield. In the event of more serious ocular injuries—such as penetration of the globe or hyphema—a shield should be employed as an interim measure to protect the eye from rubbing, pressure, and further injury prior to treatment by an ophthalmologist. The shield may consist of a perforated, malleable piece of metal **(Fig. 52)** or a trimmed-down paper cup.
- ○ Bilateral patching. Bilateral eye patching for unilateral eye trauma is of debatable benefit.
- Suturing. Suturing of any eyelid skin laceration that does not involve the eyelid margin or the lacrimal canaliculi can be performed by the primary care physician. More involved lid lacerations should be referred to an ophthalmologist.

Points to Remember

- *Point 1.* Know your limits: Do not attempt complex repair and know the results of inadequate repair.
- *Point 2.* Almost without fail, a teardrop-shaped pupil and a flat anterior chamber in an injured eye are associated with a perforating injury of the cornea or of the limbal area. Look for prolapse of dark tissue (either iris or ciliary body) at the point of the teardrop.
- *Point 3.* Penetrating injury in one eye may lead to loss of vision in the uninjured eye as a result of sympathetic ophthalmia. Actually a rare form of uveitis, sympathetic ophthalmia is a cause of such concern to ophthalmologists that a decision to enucleate an injured eye may be made after approximately one week unless there is significant return of visual function.

- *Point 4.* Vitreous hemorrhage is a common cause of sudden, painless loss of vision. Through the ophthalmoscope, the media may be clear anteriorly, but either there is no light reflex or fewer fundus details are visible. Since detachment of the vitreous is frequently a cause of hemorrhage and retinal tears, these patients often need hospital admission and observation by an ophthalmologist.

- *Point 5.* Avoid digital palpation of the globe in the patient who may have a corneal laceration or other perforating injury.

- *Point 6.* Pupillary dilation to permit evaluation of the fundus should be routine. The only exception to this general rule would be in a patient with head trauma where pupillary signs might be important for neurologic evaluation, or in patients whose shallow anterior chambers predispose them for narrow-angle glaucoma.

- *Point 7.* In a patient with a chemical burn, immediate irrigation is crucial just as soon as the nature of the injury has been learned. Do not attempt to neutralize or buffer the chemical substance. Your goal should be simply to dilute the chemical as thoroughly as possible by copious flushing.

- *Point 8.* A forceful stream of irrigating solution delivered from a squeeze bottle will often dislodge a superficial conjunctival or corneal foreign body.

Sample Problems

Multiple Choice

1. A forty-three-year-old woman is servicing her swimming pool. While pouring some concentrated algicide into the pool, a large dollop of this solution splashes into her right eye. You are mowing your lawn when you hear her screams. You come running to her aid and arrive less than thirty seconds after the injury.

   Question: Which of the following would you do first?

   (a) Bundle her into your car and speed off for the nearest emergency center.

   (b) Run back home to get your medical bag where you keep a squeeze bottle of ophthalmic irrigating solution which you can use to flush out her eye.

   (c) Run back to your study to look up the specific antidote for algicide.

   (d) Carefully examine her eye for evidence of ocular hyperemia.

   (e) Dunk her head into the swimming pool, instructing her to keep her eyes open in order to flush out the chemical.

   Answer: Choice (e). This is one of the few truly urgent situations of all the ocular injuries that you must know. Early and copious irrigation with whatever source of water is handy is the right approach to this problem. Even with prompt treatment, serious ocular injuries and visual damage may result, depending upon the offending chemical. Time is of the essence. Do not resort to methods that will cause delay.

2. You are on duty in the emergency center when an eighteen-year-old high school student comes in because of pain, tearing, sensitivity to light, and blurred vision in her right eye. Her symptoms began some time that afternoon. Earlier, she had been working on her car and she remembers something flying into her right eye while she was trying to knock a rivet off the chassis with a hammer and chisel.

You examine her eye and take visual acuity measurements. You determine that visual acuity is 20/50 in the right eye and 20/20 in the left eye. There is some conjunctival hyperemia. The pupil of the right eye seems to be peaked and pointing to the seven o'clock position of the limbus. There is a small, dark, slightly elevated body at the seven o'clock position of the limbus. You cannot see fundus details on the right, but the left eye appears normal.

Question: Which of the following would be the appropriate method of management for this situation?

(a) irrigation of the limbal foreign body

(b) application of a light patch and protective shield

(c) removal of the limbal foreign body with a cotton-tipped applicator

(d) removal of the limbal foreign body using forceps

(e) a prescription for topical anestheic (e.g., proparacaine 0.5%) to relieve the patient's symptoms, with strict instructions that she return to see you should her blurred vision continue into the week

Answer: Choice (b). Any patient whose recent activities involve striking metal on metal should be suspected of having a foreign body, even with minimal signs and symptoms. However, the case illustrated includes a giveaway sign, namely, peaking of the pupil toward the seven o'clock position. At that position, the dark body is likely to be iris or ciliary body rather than a foreign body. This indicates a penetrating ocular injury; therefore, the patient should be protected from further eye trauma by employing a light patch and a protective shield. An X ray will confirm the diagnosis of ocular or orbital foreign body. The patient should be considered an urgent referral to an ophthalmologist.

Analysis

3. While cutting his roses, a neighbor develops a sudden pain in his left eye. Inspection is limited since his eyes are closed, but nothing is visible on external examination.

Question a: What do you think might have happened?

Answer: Possibilities include: (1) a foreign body on the eye, under the lid; (2) a superficial abrasion, with the extreme sensitivity of the cornea serving as a protective mechanism; or, less likely but still possible, (3) perforation by a thorn.

Question b: What skills would you need to assess and treat this problem?

Answer: You would need to take the following steps: (1) open lids gently—never force eyelids open; instill a drop of topical anesthetic, if necessary, to facilitate examination; (2) evert lids to look for a foreign

body; (3) inspect cornea and sclera for foreign body or possible perforation; (4) remove foreign body by irrigation or with a cotton-tipped
applicator; and, lastly, (5) act on any indications for drops, ointment,
or patching.

4. While you are on duty in the emergency center, a patient is brought
   in who has been involved in a car accident. His face is bloody, especially
   around the eyes. His history is unclear.

   Question a: What would you do? What would you avoid?

   Answer: Cleanse carefully, avoiding pressure on the eye of any kind.

   Question b: While cleansing, you find a cut in the eyelid. It seems easy
   to stitch, but the lids are swollen and the patient cannot open his eye.
   What next? Do you stitch the lid?

   Answer: No, it is not an emergency. First, inspect the eye for possible
   perforation.

   Question c: If the eye is normal, how should you analyze the problem
   of the lid laceration?

   Answer: The appropriate choice of treatment depends on the level of
   damage. If only the skin is involved, you may be able to stitch the lid;
   if the laceration is full thickness, referral to an ophthalmologist is preferred; any involvement of the canaliculi requires exquisite repair in
   order to avoid a tearing problem for the rest of the patient's life—referral
   to an ophthalmologist is mandatory.

Annotated References

1. Glaucoma, lens, and anterior segment trauma, in *Basic and Clinical
   Science Course.* San Francisco, American Academy of Ophthalmology,
   1986, section 8.

   Section 8 of this eleven-volume series is an excellent summary of anterior
   segment trauma, covering general principles, burns, superficial injuries,
   blunt trauma, and perforating injuries.

2. Deutsch TA, Feller DB (eds): *Paton and Goldberg's Management of Ocular
   Injuries,* ed 2. Philadelphia, WB Saunders Co, 1985.

   Used widely by ophthalmology residents, this book contains extensive
   information useful to the student or emergency center physician who
   desires more information on serious eye trauma.

3. Newell FW: *Ophthalmology: Principles and Concepts,* ed 6. St. Louis, CV
   Mosby Co, 1986.

   Ocular injuries are summarized succinctly in Chapter 7 (Injuries of the
   Eye) of this comprehensive textbook.

4. Scheie HG, Albert DM: *Textbook of Ophthalmology,* ed 9. Philadelphia,
   WB Saunders Co, 1977.

   Chapter 17 (Ocular Injuries) covers ocular injuries and contains a useful
   table summarizing the procedure for emergency center evaluation.

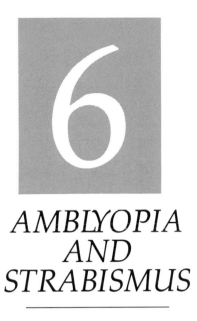

AMBLYOPIA AND STRABISMUS

Objectives

You should be able to recognize the signs and symptoms of amblyopia and strabismus; be able to perform the necessary tests to screen for these conditions; and, if the patient is a child, be cognizant of the need to arrange for prompt ophthalmological consultation, particularly when intra-ocular disease is suspected.

To achieve these objectives you should learn:

- To measure or estimate visual acuity in children.
- To detect strabismus by gross inspection, the corneal light reflex test, and the cover test.
- To perform ophthalmoscopy in a child in order to rule out organic causes of impaired vision when amblyopia is suspected.
- To explain to parents the need for prompt treatment of their child's amblyopia.

Relevance

Amblyopia is a form of treatable visual loss found in approximately two percent of the young adult population of the United States. It can be defined as a loss of visual acuity, not correctable by glasses in an otherwise normal eye. Amblyopia may be present in infancy or early childhood, and can be detected in the youngest of patients. In fact, early detection of amblyopia is the key to successful treatment. If treated early, amblyopia can be cured. Unfortunately, treatment for amblyopia is rarely successful past the age of nine years and, for best results, should begin before the age of five years. At least one half of all patients with amblyopia also have strabismus, a misalignment of the two eyes.

The pediatrician (or other primary care physician) will most likely be the first to see a young patient with amblyopia or strabismus and, therefore, will have the primary responsibility for screening. The pediatrician must be familiar with the different kinds of amblyopia and strabismus, their close relationship, and how best to test for and detect these conditions.

Basic Information

It is important to understand that vision is a developmental sensory function. Vision at birth may be relatively poor, but through proper visual stimulation in the early months and years of life, a "normal" acuity is achieved at approximately three years of age. If this developmental process—the stimulation of the vision receptive cells in the brain—is prevented because of amblyopia, strabismus, abnormal refractive error, congenital cataract, or some other condition, vision will not develop properly. This is a failure of the developmental process, not an organic abnormality of the eye.

Amblyopia

Amblyopia can be thought of as defective vision, uncorrectable by glasses, in an otherwise normal eye. Amblyopia can affect both eyes, but this is rare. Amblyopia does not have a clinically demonstrable organic basis, and it should be differentiated from those diseases that result in vision loss due to organic, ocular defects, for example, congenital cataract, retinoblastoma (a life-threatening tumor of early childhood), and other inflammatory and congenital ocular disorders. Amblyopia results in young children in whom visual information received by the brain from one eye is inadequate or conflicts with information from the other eye.

A simple way to understand the situation is to assume that the brain is receiving two stimuli for each visual event: one from a visually aligned eye and one from a "misdirected" eye. The brain selects the better image to the eventual detriment of vision in the misdirected eye. In other words, the brain continually favors the "good" eye, which results in the faulty development of vision in the amblyopic eye. For this reason, amblyopia is often referred to colloquially as "lazy eye." There are a number of predisposing factors that can lead to the development of amblyopia. These are summarized below.

Strabismic amblyopia. Amblyopia can develop in the context of strabismus. When this occurs, the two eyes are misaligned relative to each other and only one eye is looking at the object of regard. Suppression of sensory input from one eye results in the failure to develop vision in that eye, which is amblyopia. Sometimes the degree of misalignment between the two eyes may be very small, making detection difficult. Even with a small angle of strabismus, amblyopia may be quite dense.

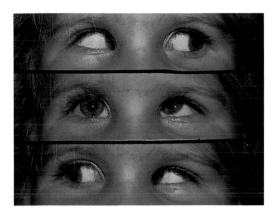

Fig. 53. Comitant (nonparalytic) strabismus. In the three views presented here, the misaligned eyes exhibit approximately the same degree of inward deviation in each position of gaze, which is characteristic of comitant strabismus.

Refractive amblyopia. Amblyopia can result from a marked difference in refractive error between the two eyes. Unequal accommodation is impossible: the child can bring only one eye at a time into focus. The eye with the lesser refractive error provides the clearer image and usually is favored over the other eye, leaving an unclear image in that eye and, again, a failure to develop vision. Refractive amblyopia may be as severe as that found in strabismic amblyopia. However, detection by the pediatrician or other primary care physician is more difficult because there is no obvious strabismus. Detection must be based on an abnormality found in visual acuity testing.

Form-deprivation and occlusion amblyopia. Form-deprivation amblyopia (amblyopia ex anopsia) can result when opacities of the ocular media, such as cataracts or corneal scarring, prevent adequate sensory input. Total sensory deprivation can be induced by prolonged patch occlusion (described later in this chapter under *Treatment*). In such cases, occlusion amblyopia can result in a previously unaffected eye.

Strabismus

Strabismus is a misalignment of the two eyes, so that both eyes cannot be directed toward the object of regard. Strabismus may be caused by the absence of binocular vision. There are a number of terms used to discuss and to classify strabismus. These are summarized below.

Comitant and Noncomitant Strabismus

It is also clinically useful to distinguish between comitant (nonparalytic) and noncomitant (paralytic or restrictive) strabismus.

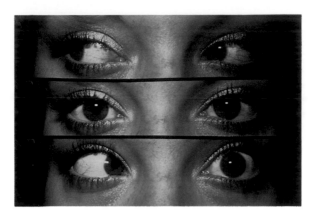

Fig. 54. Noncomitant (paralytic or restrictive) strabismus. Here the eyes appear to be fairly straight in right gaze (top) and in straight ahead gaze (middle position), but a misalignment of the eyes is obvious in left gaze (bottom), indicating a paralysis of the left lateral rectus or restriction of the left medial rectus. These eye positions would be found in a left sixth cranial nerve palsy.

Comitant (nonparalytic) strabismus. Strabismus is called comitant when the angle of misalignment is approximately equal in all directions of gaze **(Fig. 53).** The individual extraocular muscles are functioning normally but the two eyes are simply not directed towards the same target. Since most comitant strabismus has its onset in childhood, it often causes the secondary development of amblyopia (i.e., strabismic amblyopia). Nonparalytic strabismus generally is not caused by serious neurological disease under the age of six years. One has to be more concerned with the possible neurologic implications of strabismus arising later in life.

Noncomitant (paralytic or restrictive) strabismus. Strabismus is called noncomitant when the degree of misalignment varies with the direction of gaze **(Fig. 54).** One or more of the extraocular muscles or nerves is not functioning properly. This type of strabismus may well indicate either a serious neurologic disorder, such as third cranial nerve palsy *(see Chapter 7, Neuro-Ophthalmology),* or possibly orbital disease, such as the restrictive ophthalmopathy of thyroid disease or a blowout fracture.

Heterophoria and Heterotropia

Heterophoria is a latent tendency for misalignment of the two eyes which becomes manifest only if binocular vision is blocked, for instance, by covering one eye. During binocular viewing, the two eyes of a patient with heterophoria are aligned perfectly; both eyes are directed at the same object of regard. However, when one eye is covered, that eye will drift to its position of rest. Once the block is removed, the eye will realign itself with the fellow eye. Actually, a minor degree of heterophoria is normal for most individuals.

Table 6.1. Summary of Heterotropia and Heterophoria

Prefix	Name of disorder		Description
	-tropia (manifest)	-phoria (latent)	
eso-	esotropia	esophoria	inward deviation
exo-	exotropia	exophoria	outward deviation
hyper-	hypertropia	hyperphoria	upward deviation
hypo-	hypotropia	hypophoria	downward deviation

Heterotropia is really another term for strabismus. In general, "tropia" refers to a manifest deviation in which binocular vision is not possible. Some patients, however, can demonstrate an intermittent heterotropia and thus achieve binocular vision only part of the time.

Direction of the deviation. Heterophoria and heterotropia can be subdivided further in terms of the direction of the deviation involved, as summarized in **Table 6.1.**

Thus in esotropia and esophoria, the deviating eye is directed inward. Esotropia is a manifest deviation in which one eye is directed inward to some degree. It is the most common type of deviation in childhood. Esophoria is a latent inward deviation that is only apparent when binocular vision is blocked. **Illustration 6.1** depicts the different kinds of heterotropia.

Diplopia. It would seem reasonable to assume that the strabismus patient might experience double vision (i.e., diplopia) since the two eyes are not directed toward the same object. However, in most cases of comitant strabismus present in infancy and childhood, the brain learns to ignore one image; a physiologic blind spot develops in the deviated eye so that the patient does not perceive two images. While this "defense" mechanism overcomes the troublesome symptoms of diplopia, it may lead to the secondary development of amblyopia.

If a noncomitant strabismus develops after childhood in a patient with good vision, the resultant diplopia should be considered a potential indicator of serious neurologic or orbital disease. On the other hand, a comitant strabismus commonly occurs in an adult who loses most or all of the vision in one eye from intraocular disease.

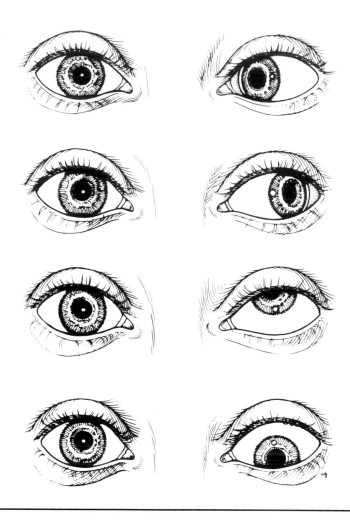

Illus. 6.1. Types of heterotropia: esotropia (inward), exotropia (outward), hypertropia (upward), and hypotropia (downward).

When to Examine

Newborn. All newborns should have the following tests: evaluation of corneal light reflex, pupillary responses, and red reflex. (The corneal light reflex test is described in the following section, *How to Examine and Interpreting the Findings. Chapter 7, Neuro-Ophthalmology,* covers pupillary responses. *Chapter 1, The Eye Examination,* describes how to evaluate the red reflex.) If retinal details can be appreciated by ophthalmoscopy, so much the better. Until three to four months of age, children often experience temporary uncoordinated eye movements and may actually exhibit intermittent strabismus during this period. However, if occasional deviation persists beyond this age, a referral to an ophthalmologist should be made. Persistent deviations should be referred at any age.

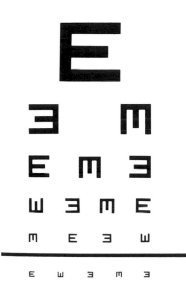

Photo 6.1.

Single E chart. Visual acuity testing in children can be done with distance charts such as the single E chart shown here.

NEAR VISION TEST

			SNELLEN PRINT SIZE	POINT SIZE
			6 M	
			3 M	27 Pt.
			2 M	18 Pt.
			1.5 M	14 Pt.
			1 M	9 Pt.
			.75 M	7 Pt.
			.5 M	5 Pt.

Photo 6.2.

Picture card. An alternative to the single E chart, this figure shows one type of picture card used to test visual acuity in young children.

Infancy. During a routine pediatric examination, the pediatrician or primary care physician should note how a child watches a light, how the eyes follow a moving object, and how the child reacts to having each eye covered in turn. The child should be able to maintain central and steady fixation with each eye. If amblyopia is present, the child will likely resent—vocally or by evasive movement—the covering of the "good" eye. Passive head movements with the infant's eyes held open can be used to demonstrate full lateral mobility, if not otherwise seen by following movements.

Age two to four years. At age three years, or younger if possible, visual acuity testing should be attempted by use of the single E chart **(Photo 6.1)** or by a picture card technique **(Photo 6.2)**. Vision should be rechecked annually once visual acuity has been determined to be normal in each eye. Young children may not quite reach 20/20 acuity. This is no cause for concern as long as both eyes are equal and vision is at least 20/40.

How to Examine and Interpreting the Findings

Amblyopia Testing

Amblyopia can be detected by testing the visual acuity in each eye separately. Although there is no specific pattern of inheritance, a family history of strabismus or amblyopia may be indicative. Restoration of normal visual acuity can be successful only if treatment occurs during the first decade of life when the visual system is still in the formative stage.

Infancy to age two years (preverbal). The examiner should note how steadily and easily the child fixates on the test object. The child should be able to follow a toy, penlight, key chain, or other highly visible target. Each eye should be tested individually while the other is covered by a hand or patch, making certain that the child cannot see around the patch. If the child consistently tries to move the blocking device from in front of one eye, then a significant vision problem may exist.

Age two years to reading age. From age two years until the child learns to read, quantitative visual acuities can be obtained for each eye by the use of picture cards (ages two to three), or the single E chart (after age three) at twenty feet or closer. To use the picture cards, the examiner familiarizes the child with the pictures at close range. Each eye is then tested individually by backing away from the child and determining the greatest distance at which the pictures can be reliably identified. The single E chart is used like the Snellen chart at twenty feet, except that the child is asked to identify with a hand gesture the direction in which the "arms" of the E are pointing. Any inequality between the vision of the two eyes or an acuity worse than 20/40 is significant.

From reading age on. Once the child can read, the conventional Snellen eye charts can be used to measure visual acuity *(see Chapter 1, The Eye Examination).*

Strabismus Testing

General inspection. A general inspection may reveal a gross deviation of one eye. Having the patient look into the cardinal positions of gaze may reveal whether or not the deviation is approximately the same in all fields of gaze—indicating comitant strabismus—or is significantly different in one field of gaze—indicating a possible noncomitant strabismus. Involuntary eye jerks known as nystagmus may be detected in primary gaze or other fields of gaze. The patient may assume an abnormal head posture (i.e., a tilt or turn to one side) to reduce the nystagmus and improve visual acuity or to obtain binocular vision in cases of congenital nerve palsy.

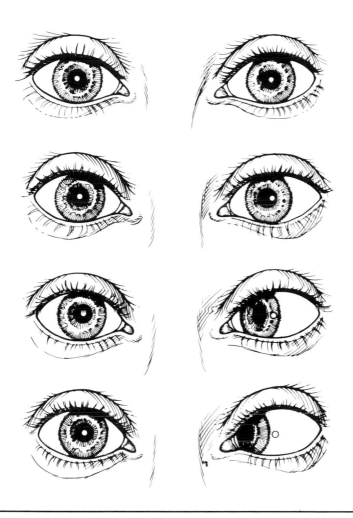

Illus. 6.2. Corneal light reflex. From top to bottom, the position of the light reflection indicates a normal alignment and a small, moderate, and large left esotropia, respectively.

Corneal light reflex. When a patient is asked to look at a penlight held by the examiner at a distance of two feet, a reflex image of the light can be seen on the cornea of the eye **(Illus. 6.2).** The examiner aligns his eye with the light source and checks for the symmetric positioning of the reflected light in relation to the pupil and visual axis of each eye. Normally, the light reflex falls at the same relative position in each eye. In a deviating eye, the light reflection will be eccentrically positioned and in a direction opposite to that of the deviation. The extent of deviation can be estimated as small, moderate, or large. In young children, this may be the only feasible method of testing for strabismus.

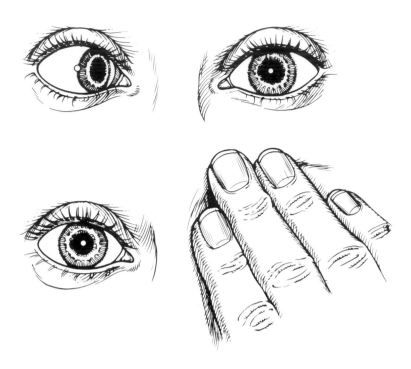

Illus. 6.3. Cover test. The cover test can be used to screen for strabismus. The results depicted here indicate a right esotropia. When the left eye is covered, the right eye moves outward to pick up fixation. (When the left eye is uncovered, the left eye moves outward to pick up fixation and both eyes assume their original positions.)

Cover test. The cover test **(Illus. 6.3)** is easy to perform, requires no special equipment, and will pick up almost every case of strabismus. To perform this test, have the patient look at a fixation point—such as a penlight or, better yet, a curiously detailed or interesting target—and note which eye seems to be the fixing eye. Cover the fixing eye and observe the fellow eye. If the uncovered eye moves to pick up the fixation, then it can be reasoned that this eye was not directed towards the object of regard originally (i.e., when both eyes were uncovered). If the eye moves inward to fixate, then originally it must have been deviated outward and hence exotropic. If the eye moves outward to pick up fixation, then it was deviated inward and is esotropic. Of course, each eye must be tested separately, since there is no way to know which eye may be expressing the deviation.

In the example shown in **Illustration 6.3,** the left eye is covered first. As it is covered, the right eye moves outward. When the right eye is covered to test the left eye, no movement of the left eye is observed. This indicates that strabismus is present (-tropia), that the right eye is the deviating eye, and that the direction of the deviation is inward (eso-). Thus, the condition is a right esotropia with a fixation preference for the left eye.

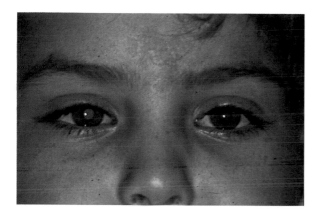

Fig. 55. Small-angle right esotropia. The corneal light reflex in the right eye is displaced very slightly to the temporal aspect of the pupil.

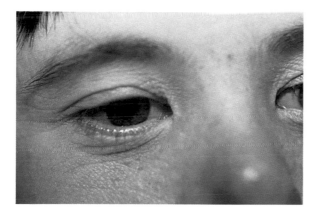

Fig. 56. Epicanthus. An extended lid fold and a relatively flat nose bridge may give the false appearance of an internal strabismus.

A very small-angle deviation **(Fig. 55)** may be difficult to detect by evaluating the corneal light reflex or performing the cover test. Visual acuity testing is very important in all cases to make certain amblyopia is not present.

Epicanthus. Infants frequently exhibit epicanthus **(Fig. 56)**, a condition in which the nose bridge is flat and skin folds extend toward the upper eyelid and brow. This gives the appearance of internal strabismus or esotropia, especially if the head or eyes are turned slightly. As the head grows and the nose bridge develops, the epicanthus becomes less obvious. This may be mistakenly interpreted as the child outgrowing the presumed strabismus. A child does not outgrow a true strabismus. The cover test and evaluation of the corneal light reflex will distinguish between epicanthus and true strabismus. However, it is important to keep in mind that strabismus can also occur in the presence of epicanthus and that the strabismus can be intermittent, apparent only when the child is tired or ill.

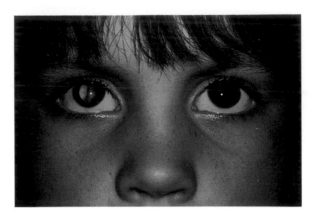

Fig. 57. Leukocoria ("white pupil"). Cataracts are not the only cause of a white reflex. In this child, a retinoblastoma fills the vitreous cavity. Any change from the normal red reflex warrants careful ophthalmic examination.

Ophthalmoscopy

A careful ophthalmoscopic examination of both eyes through dilated pupils is mandatory for any patient with reduced vision or strabismus. In this way, the examiner can detect potentially serious intraocular lesions, such as cataract or retinoblastoma, or other retinal abnormalities **(Fig. 57).**

Treatment

Treating amblyopia. In children younger than five years of age, amblyopia can usually be treated effectively by the ophthalmologist through occlusion of the unaffected eye. The child wears a patch over the "good" eye, which forces the brain to utilize the previously suppressed sensory input. In general, the success of occlusion treatment for amblyopia patients between the ages of five and nine years will depend on the age of the patient, the degree of the amblyopia, and the persistence of treatment. Treatment can be successful in children as old as ten years of age.

A treatment program started early in life often needs to be continued throughout the first decade. Amblyopia treatment by patch occlusion of the unaffected eye must be monitored carefully, especially during the younger years, to avoid causing amblyopia through sensory deprivation of the occluded eye. Treatment of refractive amblyopia consists first of wearing glasses, followed by patching of the better eye if the visual difference persists after four to eight weeks of wear. Equal vision in both eyes is readily achievable with parental cooperation. In general, the earlier the individual with amblyopia is diagnosed and treated, the better the chance of equal vision.

Correcting strabismus. The most effective way to support fusion is to treat the amblyopia and equalize the vision. Glasses can also treat the accommodative component of esotropia in a farsighted, or hyperopic, individual.

However, surgical correction of the misalignment still may be necessary. Although binocular vision may not be achievable, the impact of a disfiguring strabismus on a patient's self-image is a valid indication for surgery. It must be stressed that surgery is not an alternative for glasses and patching when amblyopia is present.

Management or Referral

The early detection of amblyopia and strabismus is extremely important for those involved in infant and child health care. Delayed diagnosis may have serious consequences in terms of visual acuity, eye disease, or systemic disease. If an abnormality is suspected, the patient should be referred promptly to an ophthalmologist. The ophthalmologist will

- first examine for intraocular disease or possible neurologic disorder;
- evaluate the need for glasses;
- institute an occlusion program if appropriate; and,
- surgically reduce the deviation if necessary.

Points to Remember

- *Point 1.* Amblyopia must be detected early in order to be treated successfully.
- *Point 2.* Amblyopia may be present in eyes without strabismus, so one cannot be confident that the vision in each eye is normal even if the eyes appear normally aligned. The importance of visual acuity testing cannot be overstressed.
- *Point 3.* Several serious organic conditions cause strabismus as one manifestation of the disease; therefore, all patients with strabismus must be referred to an ophthalmologist for further testing at the time of diagnosis.

Sample Problems

1. A three-year-old boy is brought to you by his mother who tells you that she suspects his right eye is not straight. What steps would you take to determine if a significant problem is present?

   Answer: Vision testing should be attempted using the single E chart or picture cards. A difference in visual acuity between the two eyes or decreased vision in both eyes is significant. Lastly, a suspicion of amblyopia can be investigated by observing the child's reaction to covering one eye and then the other.

   Test the alignment of the eyes by evaluating the corneal light reflex. Direct a penlight towards the child's eyes and observe the position of the light reflex. It should fall in the same position in each eye. Then proceed to the cover test. With the child still looking at the penlight, cover one eye and observe any movement of the uncovered eye. Remove the cover and then cover the other eye and observe any movement in the previously covered eye. Unequal positioning of the light reflex or movement of the uncovered eye to pick up the light fixation would suggest a misalignment of the eyes.

Perform an ophthalmoscopic examination, preferably through dilated pupils, to determine if there is any intraocular basis for visual loss, such as cataract, retinoblastoma, or a retinal abnormality.

If visual acuity is asymmetric or if there is a suspicion of intraocular disease, the patient should be referred for an urgent ophthalmologic evaluation. If visual acuity and the fundus examination are normal but strabismus is suspected because of other examination findings and/or patient history, a nonurgent referral should be made.

2. A family has just moved into your area and the mother has brought her six-month-old baby to your family practice office for a routine checkup. She mentions that the child's grandfather has noted that in several photographs the baby's left eye appears crossed. He is rather adamant in his observation and feels that "something should be done." The mother has felt that, at times, the eye has appeared crossed but the baby's father has not observed this phenomenon. How should you proceed?

Answer: Inquire about any family history of strabismus or amblyopia and observe for the presence of epicanthus. Observe the alignment of the child's eyes as you jingle your key ring. Move the key ring from side to side and up and down to assess individual muscle function. Place your hand in front of one eye and then the other to see if the child exhibits displeasure. Move the penlight through the various positions of gaze and assess the position of the corneal light reflection.

Examination reveals that significant lid folds are present. The corneal light reflex is the same in each eye, and full extraocular movements are seen in all cardinal fields of gaze. While in this case the appearance of a crossed eye is probably the result of epicanthus, continued observation on the next visit is indicated. Remember that strabismus and amblyopia can occur in a patient with epicanthus, and the strabismus may be intermittent. Any suspected abnormality should be referred to an ophthalmologist.

3. A two-year-old boy is brought to your office because his mother has noticed that over the past two weeks his right eye has deviated inward during periods of fatigue. On the previous evening, the boy's father claims to have noted a white reflex in the child's right eye. How should you proceed?

Answer: Evaluate the corneal light reflex and perform the cover test as described in the preceding problems. In particular, note whether an abnormal response is elicited on covering one eye. Test the pupillary light reflexes. Perform an ophthalmoscopic examination, preferably through a dilated pupil, to observe for organic pathology.

Examination reveals equal pupillary light reflexes. A poor red reflex is noted on ophthalmoscopic examination of the right eye as compared with the left. No detail can be seen in the right fundus. Your findings indicate the need for an urgent referral. Following ophthalmological consultation, the esotropia in this child was diagnosed as secondary to a retinoblastoma.

4. A fifty-four-year-old man has early cataracts in both eyes. With glasses, the right eye cannot be corrected to better than 20/200 visual acuity, whereas with the left eye he can read the 20/40 line with best correction. The amount of cataract is exactly the same in each eye. Examination of the optic disc and macula, pupillary reaction, color vision, retinal blood vessels, and intraocular pressure proved entirely normal in each eye. However, the right eye appears to be turned slightly inward when evaluating the corneal light reflex and the patient has not experienced diplopia. Additional questioning reveals that the patient wore a patch over one eye as a child. Why would information concerning his child-hood ocular condition be relevant in this situation?

Answer: The poor vision in the right eye may be due to a previous amblyopia. If this is the case, removal of the cataract would result in vision which would be only as good as that present during the adolescent years.

Annotated References

1. Gittinger JW Jr: *Ophthalmology: A Clinical Introduction.* Boston, Little, Brown & Co, 1984, pp 131–149.

   Provides the reader with a concise overview of strabismus and amblyopia. A short section on the anatomy and function of the extraocular muscles is particularly good.

2. Havener WH: *Synopsis of Ophthalmology,* ed 6. St. Louis, Mo, CV Mosby Co, 1984, pp 294–318.

   The strabismus chapter is very understandable for the student and the primary care physician. The important points are particularly well illustrated, adding to the ease of reading.

3. Newell FW: *Ophthalmology: Principles and Concepts,* ed 6. St. Louis, Mo, CV Mosby Co, 1986, pp 102–106, 356–370.

   A short discussion of the development of amblyopia will be beneficial to the reader. Ocular muscle function and ocular motility are presented in different areas of the textbook. Provides a good overview.

4. Scheie HG, Albert DM: *Textbook of Ophthalmology,* ed 9. Philadelphia, WB Saunders Co, 1977, pp 115–120, 332–343.

   The anatomy and function of the extraocular muscles are covered within the scope of the chapter on physiology. A very readable overview of strabismus and amblyopia is included in the pediatric ophthalmology chapter.

5. Vaughan D, Asbury T: *General Ophthalmology,* ed 11. Los Altos, Calif, Lange Medical Publications, 1986, pp 200–222.

   The chapter on strabismus is a comprehensive review of the subject and is well illustrated. The anatomy and physiology of the ocular muscles, as well as the sensory aspects of amblyopia, are included.

NEURO-OPHTHALMOLOGY

Objectives

As a primary care physician, you should be able to perform a basic neuro-ophthalmologic examination and to recognize and interpret the more common symptoms and signs of neuro-ophthalmologic disorders.

To achieve these objectives you should learn:

To examine and detect abnormalities of (1) visual acuity, (2) pupillary reactions, (3) function of the extraocular muscles, (4) peripheral vision (visual fields), and (5) the optic nerve head.

Relevance

The eye is a window to the central nervous system. Approximately thirty-five percent of the sensory fibers entering the brain are in the two optic nerves. It is estimated that sixty-five percent of intracranial diseases exhibit neuro-ophthalmological symptoms and/or signs. If a primary care physician conducts a routine neurovisual examination, he will frequently uncover some abnormality indicating that the patient has a neurological disorder. Important examples are brain tumors, multiple sclerosis, cerebrovascular atherosclerosis, and cerebral aneurysms.

Neuro-Ophthalmologic Examination

The neuro-ophthalmologic survey may be a rather simple examination calling for only a few minutes of the primary care physician's time, or may require referral to an ophthalmologist and many hours of sophisticated procedures. This chapter will address routine tests and screening procedures.

Visual acuity. The first step in any eye examination is to measure visual acuity. The chief complaint of most patients with eye problems is some aberration of vision. Measurement of visual acuity is an absolute necessity. Use of the conventional Snellen eye chart is currently the easiest and best method of measuring the function of the macular fibers. Both distance and near vision should be measured and recorded (*see Chapter 1, The Eye Examination*).

Pupils. This examination begins with inspection of the pupils, while the patient is looking in the distance to avoid the pupillary constriction that occurs with the near response. Inspection of dark brown irides will be easier with a tangentially applied light. The pupils should be round and equal in diameter. Unequal pupils must be measured, using a millimeter rule or a pupil gauge. Next, the pupillary light reflexes are tested, both the direct and the consensual reactions being noted. Ideally, this is done in dim room illumination, with a very bright light as stimulus. For a schematic of the pupillary pathways and reflexes, see **Illustrations 7.1 and 7.2.**

"The swinging flashlight test is the most valuable clinical test for optic nerve dysfunction currently available to the general physician" (Miller, 1985, p. 477; see Ref. 2 at the end of this chapter). The abnormality detected with this test is the afferent pupillary defect, also known as the Marcus Gunn pupil. (Before reading further, please refer to **Illus. 7.2** for the column labeled "Afferent Defect.") To perform the test, a dark room and a very bright light are necessary. The patient must maintain fixation on a distant object (fifteen feet or more away). The bright light is held directly in front of one eye for three to five seconds, then moved rapidly in front of the opposite eye for three to five seconds, and then shifted back to the first eye. This is repeated several times until the examiner is certain of the responses. The critical observation to be made is the behavior of the pupil when it is first illuminated. A normal response is an initial pupillary contraction followed by slow redilation. An abnormal response is a slow dilation without the initial contraction. A relative afferent pupillary defect almost always means a lesion in the optic nerve on the same side; although, occasionally, a large retinal lesion will also produce this pupil defect.

Ocular motility. Eye movements should be tested if the patient has a complaint of double vision, or if neurologic disease is suspected. The patient is asked to look straight up, then up and left, then straight left, and so forth. With some patients, the examiner will find it is easier for the patient to hold an eccentric gaze position when the examiner places his finger or a target in the direction in which the patient is requested to look. In either case, the eyelids should be held up with the examiner's finger when the patient is in down gaze so that the full excursion of the eyes can be seen. The examiner should be watching for one of two abnormalities: failure of one or both eyes to exhibit a full range of motion, or spontaneous jerking movements of the eyes, known as *nystagmus.*

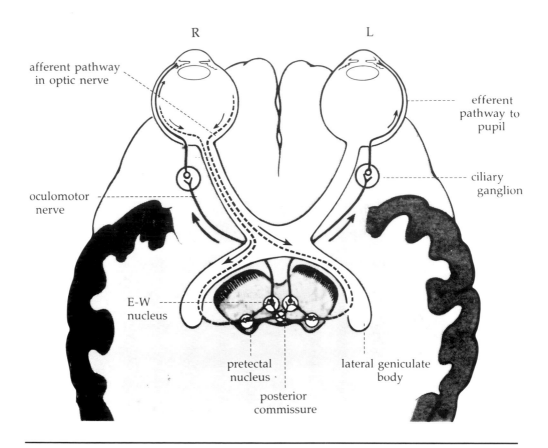

R   L

afferent pathway
in optic nerve

efferent
pathway to
pupil

ciliary
ganglion

oculomotor
nerve

E-W
nucleus

pretectal
nucleus

lateral geniculate
body

posterior
commissure

Illus. 7.1. Pupillary pathways. The view shown is a cross-section. The solid line represents the efferent pathway and the broken line represents the afferent pathway. A light stimulating the left retina will generate impulses which travel up the left optic nerve and divide at the chiasm. Some impulses continue up the left tract; some cross and continue up the right tract. The impulses arrive at each pretectal nucleus and stimulate cells, which in turn send impulses down the third cranial nerve to each iris sphincter, causing each pupil to contract. It is because of the double decussation, the first in the chiasm and the second between the pretectal nuclei and the E-N nuclei, that the direct pupil response in the left eye equals the consensual response in the right eye.

Visual fields. Evaluation of the visual fields should never be omitted from a basic eye examination. Gross confrontation testing is a satisfactory screening procedure. Each eye must be tested separately. While fixing on the examiner's eye, the patient is asked to count fingers in each of the four quadrants of the peripheral visual field. *(See Chapter 1, The Eye Examination, for additional information on confrontation testing.)* Acceptable alternate

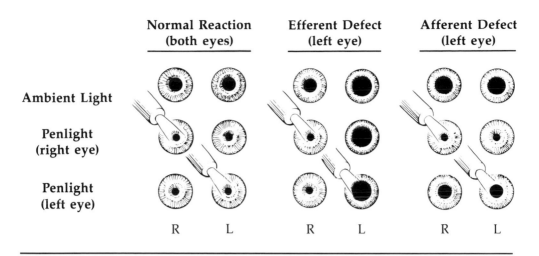

	Normal Reaction (both eyes)	Efferent Defect (left eye)	Afferent Defect (left eye)

Ambient Light

Penlight (right eye)

Penlight (left eye)

| | R L | R L | R L |

Illus. 7.2. Pupillary reflexes. As the labels indicate, the orientation depicted is that of the examiner looking at the patient's eyes.

methods include recognizing a small white pin or a similar object in all fields of vision. A red object also may be a very valuable test object in evaluating neurologic fields. Central field testing can be accomplished by means of an Amsler grid. *(See Chapter 3, Chronic Visual Loss, Photo 3.3, for figure of Amsler grid and further discussion of its use in central field testing.)*

Neuro-Ophthalmologic Symptoms and Signs

Disorders of the Pupil

Disorders of pupillary function are among the most accurate of the localizing signs of neurologic disease. Ocular disease and the influence of systemic or local drugs on the pupils must be ruled out before pupillary abnormalities can be considered to be of neurologic significance. Some of the more commonly encountered pupillary abnormalities are discussed below.

Dilated pupil. A dilated pupil, especially one that does not react to light, usually indicates a lesion in the efferent limb of the pupillary reflex (see efferent defect in **Illus. 7.2**). When a dilated pupil occurs in a patient with a head injury (or in a patient with a cloudy sensorium), it often indicates compression of the third cranial nerve (oculomotor nerve) by herniation of the temporal lobe and is of grave importance. On the other hand, a dilated, fixed pupil in an otherwise asymptomatic, healthy patient is usually innocent. In a healthy individual, a dilated pupil may reflect a benign lesion in the ciliary ganglion (a so-called tonic pupil) or may be secondary to instillation of a dilating eyedrop.

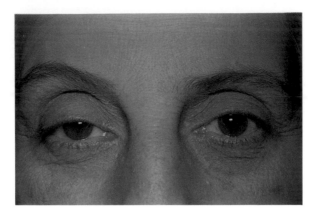

Fig. 58. Horner's syndrome. This acquired lesion of the cervical sympathetic chain has caused a mild ptosis of the right upper eyelid and a narrowing of the right pupil.

The tonic pupil. The tonic pupil, known as *Adie's pupil*, is seen predominantly in young women and is usually unilateral. In ordinary light the tonic pupil is usually larger than its counterpart; the reaction of the tonic pupil to light is either diminished or absent. Instillation of weak cholinergic agents—for example, pilocarpine hydrochloride *(Isopto® Carpine)* diluted to 0.125%—will cause constriction of a tonic pupil, whereas this concentration will not affect the normal pupil. By itself, a tonic pupil is of no neurologic significance.

A unilateral small pupil. A small pupil in one eye with normal light and near reaction is usually a physiologic anisocoria and is of no neurologic significance. However, an accompanying ptosis of the upper eyelid may indicate Horner's syndrome **(Fig. 58).** Horner's syndrome is caused by a congenital or acquired lesion of the sympathetic pathways, either in the central or preganglionic portion (from the hypothalamus to the superior cervical ganglion) or in the postganglionic portion (from the superior cervical ganglion to the eye). Detection can be accomplished through the instillation of cocaine 5 to 10%, which will dilate a normal pupil but not a Horner's pupil. Differentiation of pre- and postganglionic lesions is important and can usually be accomplished through the instillation of hydroxyamphetamine *(Paredrine®)* drops, which will dilate the pupil in a preganglionic lesion but will have no effect on a postganglionic lesion.

Diplopia

Evaluation of the patient whose complaint is double vision must include a thorough neurologically oriented history. True diplopia—which means that two separate, equally bright images are visualized, with one of the images disappearing when one eye is closed—signifies a misalignment of the visual axes of the two eyes *(see Chapter 6, Amblyopia and Strabismus).*

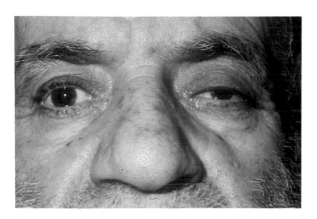

Fig. 59. Third cranial nerve paresis. This figure shows an abducted hypotropic left eye. Note the ptosis of the upper eyelid.

Patients sometimes say they are having double vision when they mean they are having blurring of vision in one eye, for example, aberration of vision in one eye due to mucous strands in the tear film. Persistence of a double image when one eye is closed indicates monocular diplopia, rather than a misalignment of the visual axes of the two eyes. It is important to note in the history whether the diplopia is transient or steady; sudden or gradual in onset; horizontal, vertical, or diagonal; and the same in all positions of gaze, or eliminated or minimized in some positions of gaze.

Neuro-Motility Disorders

Some significant neuro-motility disorders that the primary care physician should recognize are discussed below. *(It may be helpful to refer to Illus. 1.3 in Chapter 1, The Eye Examination, for a visual of the extraocular muscles.)*

Third cranial nerve paresis. Cranial nerve III (oculomotor nerve) supplies the levator palpebrae (levator muscles of the upper eyelids), the superior rectus, medial rectus, inferior rectus, and inferior oblique muscles, as well as carrying parasympathetic fibers to the sphincter of the iris. Complete paralysis of the oculomotor nerve produces both horizontal and vertical diplopia with ptosis of the upper eyelid and an inability to rotate the eye upward, inward, or downward **(Fig. 59).** The pupil may be dilated and nonresponsive. The most common causes of isolated third nerve palsy include intracranial aneurysms (especially posterior communicating aneurysms), vascular disease (including diabetes and hypertension), trauma, and brain tumor.

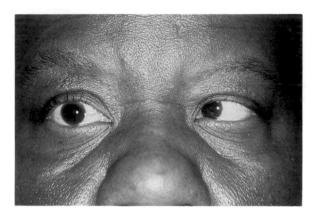

Fig. 60. Sixth cranial nerve paresis. Shown here is a complete abduction deficit of the right eye on right gaze.

Fourth cranial nerve paresis. Cranial nerve IV (trochlear nerve) innervates the superior oblique muscle so that complete paralysis causes a vertical and oblique diplopia. The patient often notices more difficulty in down gaze, and will usually tilt the head toward the opposite shoulder to minimize the diplopia. The most frequent cause of isolated fourth nerve palsy is closed head trauma, but this condition is also found in patients with vascular disease and intracranial mass lesions.

Sixth cranial nerve paresis. Cranial nerve VI (abducens nerve) supplies the lateral rectus muscle, therefore complete paralysis produces a loss of abduction and a horizontal diplopia with the greatest separation of the images when gaze is directed toward the affected side **(Fig. 60).** Intracranial tumors account for approximately thirty percent of cases of isolated sixth nerve paralysis. Head trauma, vascular disease, and increased intracranial pressure also are frequent causes of abducens paresis.

Myasthenia gravis. Myasthenia gravis is a chronic autoimmune condition that interferes with neuromuscular transmission in skeletal muscles. It can affect any muscles, but ptosis and/or double vision are the presenting signs in about one half of patients. It is characterized by fatigability of muscle function on sustained effort. Myasthenia gravis may mimic nearly any other ocular motility problem, including III, IV, and VI nerve disease, gaze paresis, and internuclear ophthalmoplegia. All patients with unexplained diplopia and/or ptosis must have an edrophonium chloride *(Tensilon®)* test.

Internuclear ophthalmoplegia. Lesions of the medial longitudinal fasciculus—an interneuron connecting the ipsilateral sixth nerve nucleus to the contralateral third nerve nucleus—are usually of considerable diagnostic significance. The clinical manifestation of such a lesion is straight eyes in primary gaze, but weakness of the adducting eye and nystagmus of the abducting eye in lateral gaze. It may be unilateral or bilateral, but convergence remains intact. In older adults, internuclear ophthalmoplegia is usually caused by vascular disease in the vertebral-basilar artery system and its terminal branches. In younger adults, it is almost always due to demyelinating disease. In children, an internuclear ophthalmoplegia calls for an MRI scan to rule out a pontine glioma, unless the child is known to have vasculitis.

Nystagmus. Spontaneous, rhythmic, back and forth movements of one or both eyes are referred to as nystagmus. Nystagmus direction may be horizontal, vertical, rotary, or combinations thereof.

The primary care physician should know that two of the most common forms of nystagmus are benign and do not indicate central nervous system dysfunction. The first type is called end-point nystagmus; it occurs when the patient is attempting to maintain his eyes in the extremes of lateral gaze. In that position, it is not unusual for the eyes to drift back slightly from the extreme horizontal gaze position, then to refixate with a small jerk movement. End-point nystagmus is usually not well sustained and disappears if the patient is permitted to move his gaze just slightly away from the extreme position. The second form of benign nystagmus is induced by drugs: diphenylhydantoin, the barbituates, and some other sedatives. The nystagmus form is identical to that seen with lesions in the vestibular system: there is a jerk nystagmus in the direction of gaze with either right or left gaze that changes to a fine upbeating nystagmus in up gaze. Often there is no nystagmus in down gaze or in straight ahead gaze. The clue to the cause of this form of nystagmus is, of course, a history of the patient's drug intake. Also, a searching, pendular nystagmus is commonly seen in congenitally blind individuals.

Almost all other forms of nystagmus are pathological, and indicate central nervous system (CNS) dysfunction. Representative diseases that cause nystagmus are multiple sclerosis, brain tumor, and CNS degenerations. Pathological nystagmus calls for referral to a specialist.

Papilledema and Optic Atrophy

Evaluation of the patient with neurologic symptoms is not complete without evaluation of the ocular fundus, with particular attention given to the appearance of the optic disc.

Elevation of the Disc

Congenital anomalous disc elevation. Occurring in slightly less than one percent of the population, congenital anomalous disc elevation is a benign, nonprogressive condition. The disc margins are blurred, the disc substance is elevated, and the cup often is obliterated, but there is no edema and no hemorrhage. Congenital disc elevation may be associated with a hyperopic refractive error, with glial tissue or persistent hyaloid remnants on the disc, or with drusen of the disc. Because of their deceptive appearance, these congenital conditions have been called pseudopapilledema **(Fig. 61).** They should not be confused with true, acquired papilledema. Such differentiation can be difficult. The diagnosis of papilledema sometimes cannot be made without evidence of progression obtained through serial examination or other diagnostic tests, such as fluorescein angiography or lumbar puncture.

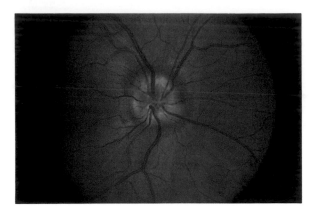

Fig. 61. Pseudopapilledema. This compact disc shows elevation and blurring of the disc margins. However, the retinal vessels appear normal, the disc is not congested, and there are no hemorrhages or other retinal abnormalities.

True papilledema. True papilledema is one of the most important ophthalmoscopic findings that the examiner must be able to recognize. Swelling of the optic disc secondary to increased intracranial pressure occurs in approximately fifty percent of patients with brain tumor. Characteristics of fully developed papilledema include hyperemia of the disc, tortuosity of the veins and capillaries, blurring and elevation of the margins of the disc, and hemorrhages on and surrounding the nerve head. The signs of early papilledema may not be quite as distinct. There may be only subtle elevation of the disc margins, separation of the nerve fibers, absence of spontaneous venous pulsation, and mild hyperemia. In addition to intracranial mass lesions, true papilledema may be seen in pseudotumor cerebri and in severe systemic hypertension.

Papillitis. Inflammatory edema of the disc, known as papillitis or anterior optic neuritis, is indistinguishable from papilledema by its ophthalmoscopic appearance. Nevertheless, the distinction is easy to make because papillitis is usually unilateral, and papilledema is usually bilateral. In addition, papillitis usually causes a dramatic reduction in visual acuity, an accompanying relative afferent pupillary defect, and distinctive alterations in the visual field, whereas such changes are not found in true papilledema. *(For a visual comparison of papillitis and papilledema, see Chapter 2, Acute Visual Loss, Figs. 10 and 11, respectively.)*

Optic Atrophy

Optic atrophy **(Fig. 62),** or pallor of the optic disc, results from damage to the nerve fiber layer of the retina, the optic nerve, optic chiasm, or optic tracts. With progressive loss of axons and alteration in glial tissue, the disc becomes less pink and more pale. After extensive damage, the disc may become chalk white. There is a wide range of physiologic pallor

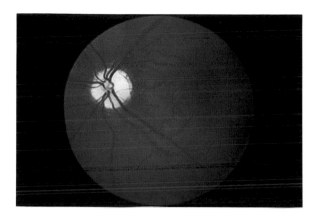

Fig. 62. Optic atrophy. This disc is flat and totally white. The sharp margins and clear definition of the disc suggest a primary disturbance of the retinal ganglion cells or their axons, rather than an inflammatory etiology at the disc.

of the disc. A diagnosis of optic atrophy should not be made unless there is decreased visual acuity or visual field loss accompanying the paleness of the disc or, if unilateral, a relative afferent pupillary defect. Common causes of optic atrophy include:

- previous optic neuritis or long-standing papilledema;
- compression of the nerve by a mass lesion, such as meningioma;
- ischemic damage to the optic nerve, namely ischemic optic neuropathy;
- optic atrophy associated with glaucoma *(see Chapter 3, Chronic Visual Loss)*.

Visual Field Defects

Visual field terminology. In summary, the following terms are commonly used to discuss visual field loss.

- scotoma: an area of reduced or absent vision within the visual field.
- hemianopia: loss of one half of the visual field. Usually involves loss of either the right or left half of the field; however, the term altitudinal hemianopia may signify loss of the superior or inferior half of the visual field.
- homonymous hemianopia: loss of either the right or left half of the visual field in both eyes.
- bitemporal hemianopia: loss of the right half of the visual field in the right eye and the left half of the visual field in the left eye.

Lesions anywhere in the visual system, from the retina to the occipital lobes, will produce visual field defects **(Illus. 7.3)**. Although detection and

Visual Pathways

Associated Field Defects

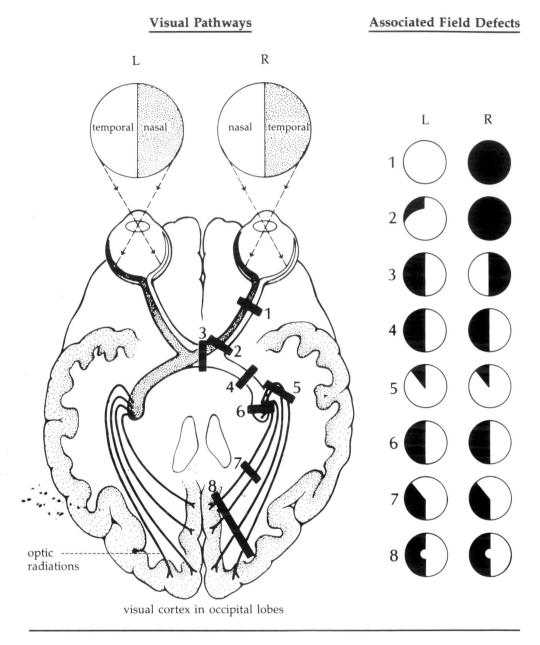

L   R

temporal   nasal   nasal   temporal

1

3
2

4   5

6

7

8

optic
radiations

visual cortex in occipital lobes

L   R

1

2

3

4

5

6

7

8

Illus. 7.3. Visual pathways with associated field defects. For the visual pathways, the view shown is a cross-section seen from above. Note that objects in the right half of the visual field form images in the left half of each retina and are transmitted to the left hemisphere. The numbers correspond to lesions in the visual pathways and to the field defects that result from these interruptions. For the purposes of the diagram, the fields shown reflect the effects of total interruption of the indicated structures. In actuality, partial impairment is more the rule than the exception. A key follows, indicating the site of each lesion and the associated field defect.

	Site of lesion	Associated field defect
1	Optic nerve	Monocular loss of vision
2	Optic nerve merging with chiasm	Monocular loss of vision associated with contralateral impairment of temporal field
3	Optic chiasm	Bitemporal hemianopia
4	Optic tract	Total homonymous hemianopia — *opthalmic migraines* (usually noncongruous if incomplete)
5	Temporal lobe	Upper homonymous hemianopia
6	Geniculate body	Rare total homonymous hemianopia
7	Parietal lobe	Lower homonymous quadrantanopia
8	Occipital lobe	Variety of homonymous hemianopias, ranging from total to small homonymous scotomas, depending on portion of lobe involved. High degree of congruity (i.e., correspondence of the field defects in the two eyes).

analysis of these field defects have led to entire texts written on the science of perimetry, most physicians need only be concerned with a few types of visual field loss. Neurologically significant field defects are most often either central scotomas (e.g., optic nerve lesions), bitemporal field defects (e.g., lesions in the region of the optic chiasm), or homonymous field defects (e.g., retrochiasmal pathways: the optic tracts, the radiations, or the occipital cortex).

Lesions in front of the chiasm. Lesions anterior to the chiasm—namely, lesions in the optic nerve—produce field defects in one eye only. Optic nerve dysfunction typically causes a central scotoma with an accompanying reduction in visual acuity.

Lesions in the optic chiasm. These lesions produce field defects that affect both eyes, but in a dissimilar fashion. The most common example is bitemporal hemianopia. Another common defect is a loss of central field in one eye accompanied by a temporal field defect in the opposite eye.

Lesions affecting the visual pathways behind the chiasm. These lesions produce homonymous hemianopias, or homonymous defects that are less than a complete hemianopia. Because the fibers serving corresponding portions of the two retinas lie increasingly closer together as the fibers pass backward toward the occipital cortex, there is greater correspondence of the field defects in the two eyes as lesions occur more posteriorly. Central visual acuity is not affected in homonymous hemianopias unless both hemispheres are involved.

Sample Problems

1. A forty-five-year-old woman comes to the emergency center because of severe left-sided headache and double vision that began the night before, immediately following sexual intercourse. As you examine her, she continues to complain of severe left-sided headache. You observe all aspects of her neuro-ophthalmological examination to be normal, except for the following: (1) the left upper lid is ptotic (drooped); (2) the left eye is deviated outward and fails to elevate, depress, or adduct normally; (3) the left pupil is dilated three millimeters more than the right and responds very poorly to light, both directly and consensually. What is your differential diagnosis? How would you proceed with evaluation and management?

    Comment: The findings are those of a left third nerve palsy with involvement of the pupil. The features of this case, including age and sex of the patient, suddenness of onset, accompanying headache, and the fact that onset occurred in conjunction with sexual intercourse, are presented to raise the issue of a possible berry aneurysm of the circle of Willis. All of the preceding factors are commonly observed in acutely expanding aneurysms arising at the junction of the internal carotid and posterior communicating arteries. Such an aneurysm is the most common cause of third nerve palsy with pupillary involvement. Interestingly, expanding aneurysms that impair cranial nerve function involve the third nerve more frequently than the other cranial nerves. Even though the patient may have no symptoms other than headache and those symptoms caused by the third nerve palsy, a symptomatic aneurysm must be suspected until proved otherwise. This is one of the true emergencies with which an ophthalmologist deals. The management in this case calls for an immediate neurosurgical referral.

In the above situation, the pupil was dilated. If the same patient appeared with exactly the same findings except for a normal left pupil, the diagnosis and management would be different. A pupil-sparing third nerve palsy most likely is due to diabetes or to some other microvascular obstruction causing ischemia of the core of the oculomotor nerve. Therefore, a pupil-sparing third nerve palsy is not a neurosurgical emergency, and the patient should be worked up for diabetes, giant-cell arteritis, syphilis, etc.

2. A twenty-five-year-old medical student suddenly complains of horizontal diplopia. Her eyes are straight when looking directly ahead, but when she attempts to look to the right or left, the eye which ought to adduct fails to move normally. However, when asked to look at the examiner's finger at a distance of six inches, both eyes converge normally. The only abnormality is vertical nystagmus when she looks up. What is the neuro-anatomic localization of this problem? What is the etiologic diagnosis?

Comment: The description is that of bilateral internuclear ophthalmoplegia. The medial longitudinal fasciculi conduct impulses to those third cranial nerve nuclei essential for participation in horizontal gaze movements. Acute, bilateral impairment of function of the medial longitudinal fasciculi occurring in this age group is typical of multiple sclerosis.

3. A thirty-two-year-old female geologist has noticed slowly progressive blurring of vision for about one month. She visited an optometrist in a shopping center and he changed her glasses, but the new glasses only helped a little. After the symptoms had been present for three months, she visited her family doctor, who found nothing wrong and referred her to a neurologist. The neurologist told her he could find no abnormality and suggested she might possibly be suffering from stress. She now comes to see you because, although she is under considerable stress, her vision keeps getting more blurred. You conduct a basic eye examination and find the following: visual acuity in the left eye is 20/60 and does not improve with a pinhole lens; the swinging flashlight test discloses a left relative afferent pupillary defect; a confrontation visual field test suggests a temporal defect in the left eye only; and there is equivocal pallor of the left optic disc. What is the differential diagnosis? Is additional testing required or should this patient be followed further?

Comment: The history of slowly progressive visual loss and the presence of a Marcus Gunn pupil virtually prove that the patient has a left optic nerve lesion. Optic neuritis is a possibility, but it usually produces sudden onset of visual loss, with recovery after a few weeks or months. The history and the findings are strongly suggestive of a tumor compressing the left optic nerve. Detailed visual field testing will probably reveal a major field defect in the left eye and a normal field in the right eye.

This localizes the lesion to the prechiasmal optic nerve, either in the orbit or in the brain. A CT scan or an MRI scan would be the logical test to order next, with the expectation that it will show a meningioma or another kind of mass compressing the optic nerve.

Annotated References

1. Burde RM, Savino PJ, Trobe JD: *Clinical Decisions in Neuro-Ophthalmology.* St. Louis, Mo, CV Mosby Co, 1985.

   Algorithmic approach to neuro-ophthalmology. A concise review of current management of neuro-ophthalmic problems. Excellent photographs and flow charts.

2. Miller NR: *Walsh & Hoyt's Clinical Neuro-Ophthalmology,* ed 4. Baltimore, Md, Williams & Wilkins, 1982, vol 1; 1985, vol 2.

   This two-volume set is the complete reference for clinical neuro-ophthalmology—the encyclopedia on the subject. Invaluable to both student and clinician.

3. Miller NR: The ocular fundus in neuroophthalmology, in Fine SL (ed): *Sights and Sounds in Ophthalmology.* St. Louis, Mo, CV Mosby Co, 1977, vol 3.

   This slide-tape set consists of a valuable collection of fundus slides with a clear discussion of the clinical and pathologic significance of retinal and optic nerve changes.

4. Walsh TJ: *Neuro-ophthalmology: Clinical Signs and Symptoms,* ed 2. Philadelphia, Lea & Febiger, 1985.

   A good general text with a clinical focus. Chapters are headed by signs and symptoms to facilitate students'understanding. Discussions are concise and clear.

OCULAR
MANIFESTATIONS
OF SYSTEMIC DISEASE

Objectives

This chapter discusses the ocular manifestations of systemic disease. Diabetes mellitus is emphasized as an important example of a systemic disease that may have serious ocular manifestations: diabetic retinopathy. As a primary care physician, you should be able to recognize and classify the three stages of diabetic retinopathy and to determine when the patient requires referral to an ophthalmologist for consultation and treatment. In addition, you should become familiar with the ocular findings associated with systemic hypertension, thyroid disease, sarcoidosis, acquired immune deficiency syndrome, and herpes zoster ophthalmicus.

To achieve these objectives you should learn:

- To measure the visual acuity of the diabetic patient *(see Chapter 1, The Eye Examination, for the measurement of visual acuity)*.
- To recognize on ophthalmoscopic examination the characteristic features of nonproliferative, preproliferative, and proliferative diabetic retinopathy.
- When to refer a diabetic patient to an ophthalmologist.

Relevance

Diabetic retinopathy is one of the four most frequent causes of newly diagnosed blindness in the United States, and the leading cause in the twenty to sixty-four year age group. Treatment of diabetic retinopathy is geared toward the prevention of visual loss. Preventative treatment is often indicated even when the diabetic has good vision and is unlikely to consult an ophthalmologist. By including careful ophthalmoscopic examinations in the routine care of the diabetic patient, the primary care physician can screen for the twenty-five percent of the diabetic population who have diabetic retinopathy and refer those patients who need the consultation and treatment of an ophthalmologist. In addition, he can reassure the majority of his diabetic patients that their vision is normal and that they do not have retinopathy.

Basic Information

Diabetic retinopathy is classified in three stages based on ophthalmoscopic appearance. The longer a patient suffers from diabetes, the greater the likelihood of developing diabetic retinopathy. The prevalence is seven percent in patients with diabetes for less than ten years, twenty-five percent in patients with diabetes for ten to fourteen years, and sixty-five percent in patients with diabetes for fifteen years or more.

Stage 1: Nonproliferative diabetic retinopathy (NPDR). NPDR **(Fig. 63),** also called background retinopathy, is characterized by microaneurysms, dot and blot hemorrhages, and hard exudates **(Fig. 64).** All patients diagnosed as having background retinopathy should be referred to an ophthalmologist for follow-up. If visual acuity is normal, patients in this stage of retinopathy require only observation by an ophthalmologist as opposed to treatment. Unfortunately, abnormal retinal vascular permeability in NPDR can result in edema of the macula, which is the most common cause of decreased vision in diabetic retinopathy. Patients whose vision is reduced by macular edema may be candidates for laser therapy.

Stage 2: Preproliferative diabetic retinopathy. The preproliferative stage of diabetic retinopathy is characterized clinically by cotton-wool spots (i.e., microinfarctions of the retina, **Fig. 65**), an ophthalmoscopic hallmark of retinal ischemia. Other features of the preproliferative stage **(Fig. 66)** are venous beading (irregularities in the caliber of the vein), large blot retinal hemorrhages, and widespread intraretinal microvascular abnormalities called telangiectasias (i.e., a proliferation of capillaries on the retinal surface; similar to telangiectasias of the skin). This is an important stage for the primary care physician to recognize because fifty percent of diabetics with preproliferative retinopathy will progress to the proliferative stage within twelve to twenty-four months. All patients with preproliferative retinopathy should be referred immediately to an ophthalmologist.

Stage 3: Proliferative diabetic retinopathy. The proliferative stage of retinopathy **(Fig. 67)** is characterized by new vessel growth that occurs on the optic disc and/or retina. The new vessels occur as a response to ischemia of the retina, but instead of growing into the areas of ischemic retina, they grow into the vitreous. Several complications may result.

- *Hemorrhage.* The new vessels are extremely fragile and have a tendency to bleed. Hemorrhage is often so extensive that it can fill the vitreous cavity with blood, severely obscuring vision, and occasionally resulting in permanent scar tissue formation.

- *Retinal detachment.* The neovascular tissue is composed of fibrous tissue in addition to vessels. The fibrous tissue can contract, producing traction on the retina and possible detachment, ultimately drawing the retina into scarred folds.

- *Vision Loss.* Either of the above complications can eventually result in total loss of vision.

Once traction retinal detachment has occurred, the visual prognosis is poor. Extensive and complex vitreous and retinal surgery is required; however, despite treatment, less than ten percent of patients attain reading visual acuity.

Accordingly, treatment goals at the proliferative stage of diabetic retinopathy are the prevention of vitreous hemorrhage and traction retinal detachment. In order to achieve these goals, therapy with laser photocoagulation is initiated immediately upon diagnosis of the condition, even if visual acuity is normal. Panretinal laser photocoagulation consists of scattering laser burns **(Fig. 68)** throughout the peripheral retina, sparing the retina immediately surrounding the macula. Laser photocoagulation causes regression of existing neovascular tissue and prevents future new vessel growth. When patients with proliferative diabetic retinopathy are treated early, before complications have developed, the rate of severe visual loss decreases five-fold in comparison to stage 3 patients treated later in the course of the disease.

When to Examine

Visual acuity measurement and ophthalmoscopic examination of the ocular fundi should be done twice each year for diabetic patients.

How to Examine

Distance visual acuity can be measured using a Snellen eye chart *(see Chapter 1, The Eye Examination).* In order to perform an adequate examination of the fundus, pupillary dilation is necessary. Dilate the pupils with tropicamide 1% *(Mydriacyl®)* and carefully examine the posterior pole with the direct ophthalmoscope, checking for hemorrhages, exudates, cotton-wool spots, irregular caliber of the veins, and neovascularization.

Interpreting the Findings

If visual acuity is normal and none of the findings discussed under *Basic Information* is present, the diabetic patient can be reassured that he does not have retinopathy.

If the visual acuity is abnormal, possible causes include induced myopia from lens swelling, cataract, diabetic optic neuropathy, and macular edema or vitreous hemorrhage due to diabetic retinopathy. Your examination can eliminate many of these possible diagnoses, but ophthalmoscopic findings

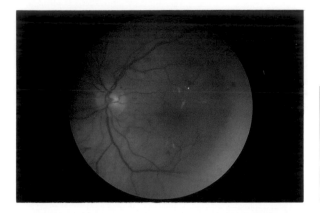

Fig. 63. Nonproliferative (background) diabetic retinopathy. Dot and blot hemorrhages and exudates are shown scattered throughout the posterior pole. Microaneurysms (pinpoint dots) are difficult to see without high magnification.

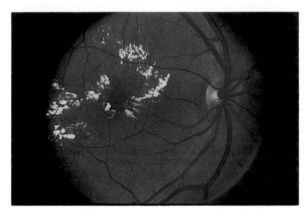

Fig. 64. Exudates. Clusters of hard, yellowish exudates within the macula are prominent in this patient with nonproliferative diabetic retinopathy.

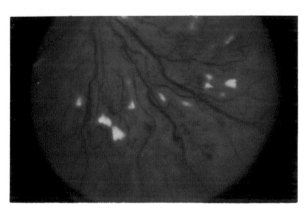

Fig. 65. Cotton-wool spots in preproliferative diabetic retinopathy. Microinfarctions of the nerve fiber layer (cytoid bodies) produce the ophthalmoscopically visible lesions shown. Cotton-wool spots are opaque white, have feathery borders, and obscure the underlying retinal blood vessels. Venous beading and telangiectasias of the retinal vasculature are shown.

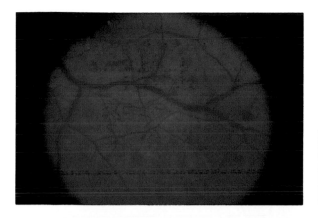

Fig. 66. Preproliferative diabetic retinopathy. Venous beading, intraretinal microvascular abnormalities, and dot and blot hemorrhages are shown.

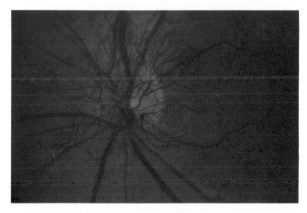

Fig. 67. Proliferative diabetic retinopathy. Shown here is a network of new blood vessels branching on the optic disc.

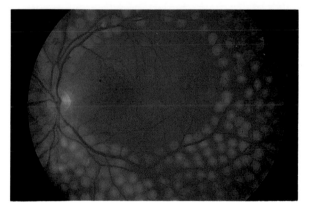

Fig. 68. Panretinal argon laser photocoagulation. This figure shows recently placed argon laser burns in the posterior pole of a diabetic patient with proliferative retinopathy. The retina immediately surrounding the macula was not treated. Over time, the laser burns develop variable pigmentation as a result of chorioretinal scarring.

may be normal in the case of diabetic optic neuropathy. If induced myopia is the cause, visual acuity will improve with the use of a pinhole during visual acuity testing *(see Chapter 1, The Eye Examination)*.

The presence of retinal hemorrhages and exudates indicates nonproliferative retinopathy; cotton-wool spots and/or venous beading indicate preproliferative retinopathy; and neovascularization and/or vitreous hemorrhage indicate proliferative retinopathy.

Management or Referral

The following guidelines can be used to determine when a diabetic patient should be referred to an ophthalmologist.

- *Type 1 diabetes.* Since type 1 diabetics typically do not develop retinopathy for at least five years after the diagnosis of diabetes, these patients generally need not be referred until five years after initial onset.

- *Type 2 diabetes.* Type 2 diabetics may have significant disease when first diagnosed, due in part to the lag time that frequently occurs between the onset of the disease and its diagnosis. These patients should have an ophthalmologic evaluation at the time of their initial diagnosis.

- *Frequency of follow-up.* The frequency of follow-up examinations by an ophthalmologist is determined by several factors but, in particular, by the stage of disease present. While a yearly examination is sufficient for some patients, others must be seen on a monthly or bimonthly basis. More frequent visits are required for patients with preproliferative disease or vitreous hemorrhages, and for diabetic patients who are undergoing laser photocoagulation for their retinopathy. During pregnancy, some diabetic patients may require more frequent monitoring by an ophthalmologist.

- *Interval referrals.* Interval referrals should be prompted by two factors: ophthalmoscopic findings and the patient's ocular symptoms. Whenever there is any ophthalmoscopic indication of a new diagnosis of proliferative tissue or vitreous hemorrhage, the patient should be referred to an ophthalmologist immediately. A patient who experiences a persistent decrease in vision or the onset of new floaters also requires immediate referral. Floaters are fine opacities in the vitreous which cast a shadow on the retina. The patient may note these as "spots," "cobwebs," "threads," or other configurations. The onset of new floaters in a patient with diabetic retinopathy often represents a vitreous hemorrhage.

Other Important Conditions

Hypertensive Retinopathy

In order to understand the effects of systemic hypertension on the retinal vasculature, it is helpful to divide hypertensive retinopathy into two classifi-

Table 8.1. Scheie Classification*

Hypertension

Grade 1:   Slight generalized attenuation of retinal arterioles

Grade 2:   Obvious arteriolar narrowing with focal areas of attenuation

Grade 3:   Grade 2 plus hard exudates, cotton-wool spots, and hemorrhages

Grade 4:   Grade 3 plus optic nerve edema

Arteriolar Sclerosis

Grade 1:   Broadening of arteriolar light reflex; minimal A/V crossing changes

Grade 2:   Obvious broadening of arteriolar light reflex and A/V crossing changes

Grade 3:   Copper-wire arterioles and more marked A/V crossing changes

Grade 4:   Silver-wire arterioles and severe A/V crossing changes

---

* *Other classifications such as the Keith-Wegener-Barker grouping do exist. Not all ophthalmologists agree on the usefulness of classifications of hypertensive changes.*

cations **(Table 8.1):** those changes due to arteriolar sclerosis and those due to elevated blood pressure.

Arteriolar Sclerosis

Although aging does cause thickening and sclerosis of the arterioles, prolonged systemic hypertension (usually diastolic pressure greater than 100 mm Hg) speeds up this process. Thickening of the walls of the retinal arterioles results in the ophthalmoscopic features of retinal arteriolar sclerosis. The amount of arteriolar sclerosis depends on the duration and severity of the hypertension and may reflect the condition of the arterioles elsewhere in the body.

Changes in the light reflex of the arteriole. In a normal eye, the retinal arterioles are transparent tubes with blood visible inside. With ophthalmoscopy, a light streak is reflected from the convex wall of the arteriole. As arteriolar sclerosis causes thickening and fibrosis of the vessel wall, the central light reflex increases in width **(Fig. 69).** After further sclerosis, the light reflex occupies most of the width of the vessels; at this point, the vessels are called copper-wire arterioles. As fibrosis continues, the light reflex is obscured totally and the arterioles appear as whitish tubes; these vessels are referred to as silver-wire arterioles.

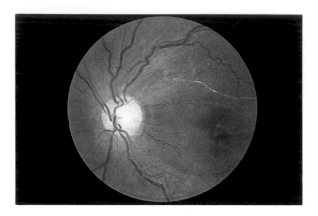

Fig. 69. Hypertensive retinopathy. A single vessel with areas of copper-wiring and silver-wiring is visible in this fundus photograph of a patient with longstanding chronic hypertension.

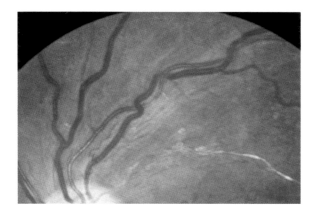

Fig. 70. Arteriovenous (A/V) crossing changes. In this magnified view of Fig. 69, an abrupt right-angle change of a vein is visible at the first AV crossing, and nicking of the vein is seen at the second AV crossing.

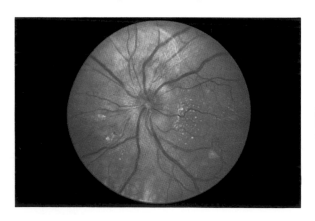

Fig. 71. Malignant hypertension. This figure depicts the ocular findings associated with severe hypertension: optic disc swelling comparable to that of papilledema, hemorrhages, exudates, and cotton-wool spots.

Arteriovenous (A/V) crossing changes. Because the arterioles and veins share a common tunnel within the retinal tissue where they cross, arteriovenous crossing changes **(Fig. 70)** can be seen. There may be zones of concealment where the vein is hidden in the region that underlies the artery. The concealment appears as narrowing, or so-called nicking, of the vein as it fades on either side of the arteriole.

The vein may be elevated or depressed by the arteriole and, in more severe cases, may undergo an abrupt right-angle change in course just as it reaches the arteriole **(see Fig. 70).** Changes in the caliber of the vein may occur because of compression and constriction at the A/V crossing, resulting in dilation of the distal portion of the vein. All of the above A/V crossing changes are most significant when found at or beyond the second bifurcation of the arteriole, which occurs about one disc diameter distant from the optic nerve head.

Hypertension

A moderate, acute rise in blood pressure results in constriction of the arterioles. A severe, acute rise in blood pressure (usually diastolic pressure greater than 120 mm Hg) causes fibrinoid necrosis of the vessel wall, resulting in exudates, cotton-wool spots, flame-shaped hemorrhages, and sometimes whitish swelling and edema of large portions of the retina. In the most severe situation of malignant hypertension **(Fig. 71),** optic disc swelling occurs which resembles that seen in papilledema.

Diagnostic Concerns

The changes due to an acute rise in blood pressure are best seen and sometimes only seen on normal arterioles, in other words, those not affected by arteriolar sclerosis, since the thickening and fibrosis of the vessel walls protect against fibrinoid necrosis. For instance, arteriolar sclerosis might mask hypertensive changes in a young patient with a pheochromocytoma or in a pregnant woman with toxemia.

It is sometimes difficult to differentiate chronic hypertensive vascular changes (i.e., arteriolar sclerosis) from normal involutional (i.e., age-related) changes. In order of importance, the most sensitive ophthalmoscopic indicators of hypertension are attenuation of the retinal arterioles, focal narrowing, and A/V crossing changes. To further complicate the diagnosis, arteriolar sclerosis and acute hypertension changes may coexist in the same patient.

Thyroid Disease

Graves' disease is an example of an important autoimmune disease that may have ocular manifestations. A common clinical feature of thyroid eye disease is retraction of the lower and/or upper eyelids, with upper lid lag on down gaze. Thyroid eye disease is also the most common cause of unilateral or bilateral protrusion of the globes, or exophthalmos, in the

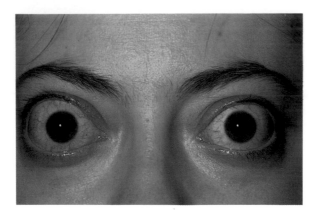

Fig. 72. Thyroid stare. The staring appearance of this patient is due to forward protrusion of the eyes and retraction of the eyelids to show white sclera above and below the limbus.

adult population. Exophthalmos in combination with retraction of the lids may produce an appearance referred to as *thyroid stare* **(Fig. 72).** Both of the above conditions result in corneal exposure and drying; this may cause the patient to complain of foreign body sensation and tearing. These symptoms are bothersome to the patient but usually can be relieved by the frequent application, sometimes hourly, of over-the-counter artificial tear preparations. The eyelid edema and conjunctival vascular congestion that sometimes accompany thyroid eye disease do not require treatment.

Thyroid eye disease may cause more serious complications requiring an ophthalmologist's care. Double vision, or diplopia, due to extraocular muscle involvement may require complicated strabismus surgery. Rarely, compression of the optic nerve within the orbit causes loss of vision, necessitating surgery to decompress the orbit.

Sarcoidosis

Sarcoidosis is a chronic, inflammatory disease that affects several organ systems. Ocular manifestations are characterized histologically by the presence of focal, noncaseating granulomas. Sarcoidosis is most common in black women of twenty to forty years of age. Diagnostic tests include:

- serum calcium: elevated in twelve percent
- anergy: present in fifty percent
- angiotensin-I-converting enzyme above 40 units: abnormal in seventy-five percent
- chest X ray: abnormal in eighty percent

The diagnosis is best confirmed histopathologically by a positive biopsy of either conjunctiva, lacrimal gland, or lymph node. Conjunctiva and lacrimal gland biopsies are easily performed in the ophthalmologist's office, using local anesthesia. Since trauma is minimal, such biopsies are usually performed before attempting more risky and invasive lymph node biopsy.

Ocular involvement may be "silent" or symptomatic; therefore, all patients suspected of sarcoidosis should be referred for a complete ophthalmologic evaluation. Early initiation of topical or systemic corticosteroids is the most effective treatment. Ocular manifestations are uveitis, retinitis, and kerato-conjunctivitis sicca.

Uveitis. Sarcoidosis may cause anterior and/or posterior uveitis. Anterior uveitis refers to inflammation of the iris and ciliary body, and posterior uveitis refers to inflammation of the choroid. If treatment is delayed, adhesions of the iris to the lens, glaucoma, and cataract may result. Uveitis can be asymptomatic.

Retinitis. Involvement of the retina is usually associated with a posterior uveitis and may present with perivasculitis, hemorrhages, and neovascularization of the peripheral retina. Involvement of the central nervous system is twice as common when the fundus is involved; in fact, the incidence doubles, increasing from ten to fifteen percent to between twenty and thirty percent.

Keratoconjunctivitis sicca. Involvement of the lacrimal gland may result in severe dry eye syndrome, requiring extensive tear replacement therapy.

Acquired Immune Deficiency Syndrome

Acquired immune deficiency syndrome (AIDS) is a severe disorder in which depression of a patient's cellular immune system results in the development of multiple opportunistic infections and Kaposi's sarcoma. Ophthalmological examination may help confirm the diagnosis. Ocular manifestations fall into three groups: (1) cotton-wool spots, (2) cytomegalovirus retinitis, and (3) Kaposi's sarcoma.

Cotton-wool spots. Retinal cotton-wool spots **(Fig. 73)** are microinfarctions of the retina indicative of retinal ischemia due to compromise of the end-arterioles. They are frequently the sole ocular finding in patients with AIDS.

Cytomegalovirus (CMV) retinitis. CMV retinitis **(Fig. 74)** is the leading cause of visual loss in patients with AIDS. It has a distinctive ophthalmoscopic appearance, characterized by hemorrhagic necrosis of the retina. Areas of involved retina have distinct borders and abruptly abut areas of normal retina. The disease progresses over weeks to months and results in total atrophy of the affected retina.

Kaposi's sarcoma. Kaposi's sarcoma, characterized by multiple vascular skin malignancies, may involve the conjunctiva of either the lid or globe. Unless suspected, it may be misdiagnosed as a hemorrhage or hemangioma.

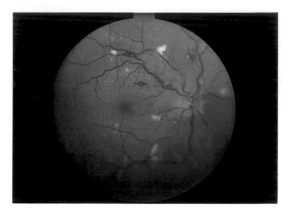

Fig. 73. Cotton-wool spots in AIDS. Scattered cotton-wool spots, as well as some hemorrhages, are depicted in this fundus photograph of a patient with AIDS.

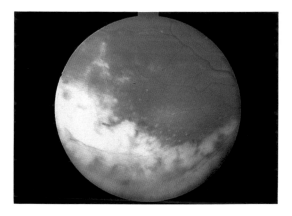

Fig. 74. Cytomegalic inclusion disease retinitis in AIDS. CMV retinitis in a patient with AIDS is shown. The retinitis is characterized by a discrete, fluffy, white retinal necrosis, with retinal hemorrhages and vasculitis. There is a sharp, distinct border between the diseased retina and the normal retina.

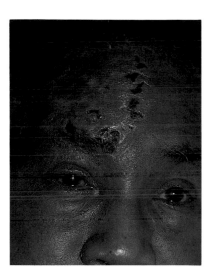

Fig. 75. Herpes zoster ophthalmicus. Crusting lesions (no longer vesicles) are present in the distribution of the ophthalmic division of the fifth cranial nerve. The conjunctiva is red and the lids are swollen, indicating ocular involvement by herpes zoster.

Herpes Zoster Ophthalmicus

Herpes zoster ophthalmicus **(Fig. 75)**, meaning herpes zoster involving the ophthalmic division of the fifth cranial nerve, may result in ocular manifestations, especially when vesicles appear on the tip of the nose (i.e., nasociliary branch). Staining of the cornea with fluorescein dye *(see Chapter 1, The Eye Examination)* may reveal corneal epithelial involvement, but examination to rule out uveitis is best performed using a slit lamp. Because herpes zoster ophthalmicus with ocular involvement is always serious and can be blinding, these patients should be referred to an ophthalmologist for examination and treatment.

Sample Problems

1. A patient with a ten-year history of adult-onset, insulin-dependent diabetes comes to your office for the first time, having recently moved from another state. She tells you that she has never seen an ophthalmologist nor had a dilated ophthalmoscopic examination. Her visual acuity is normal but on dilated fundus examination, you find neovascularization of the optic disc. How do you manage this patient?

   Comment: Although this patient's visual acuity is normal, neovascularization of the optic disc is diagnostic of proliferative diabetic retinopathy, which places this patient at serious risk of developing complications that could lead to marked visual loss. She should be referred immediately to an ophthalmologist for examination and treatment. Panretinal laser photocoagulation can be initiated to achieve regression of the neovascularization and prevent serious visual loss.

2. A forty-five-year-old man comes to your office complaining of headaches and nosebleeds. His blood pressure is 180/120 mm Hg. On dilated fundus examination, you find numerous exudates, flame-shaped hemorrhages, cotton-wool spots, and severe attenuation of the arterioles. You do not find A/V crossing changes, and the arteriolar light reflex is normal. What information does your ophthalmoscopic examination provide about the chronicity of his systemic hypertension?

   Comment: Flame-shaped hemorrhages and cotton-wool spots are ophthalmoscopic changes indicative of acute, severe hypertension. When these features occur in the absence of arteriolar sclerotic changes (i.e., A/V crossing phenomenon), hypertension is severe and most likely of recent onset; hypertension in such cases may be associated with renal insufficiency, encephalopathy, and impairment of cardiac function.

Annotated References

1. Diabetic Retinopathy Study Research Group: Photocoagulation treatment of proliferative diabetic retinopathy: The second report of diabetic retinopathy study findings. *Ophthalmology* **85**:82–106, 1978.

   A report of the findings in this classic prospective, randomized, multicenter study on diabetic retinopathy.

2. Palestine AG, Rodrigues MM, Macher AM, et al: Ophthalmic involvement in acquired immunodeficiency syndrome. *Ophthalmology* **91**:1092–1099, 1984.

   One of the best summaries of the ophthalmic changes associated with acquired immunodeficiency syndrome.

3. Retina and vitreous, in *Basic and Clinical Science Course.* San Francisco, American Academy of Ophthalmology, 1986, section 4, pp 13–22.

    These nine pages give one of the most succinct and clear descriptions of diabetic and hypertensive retinopathy available.

4. Scheie HG: Evaluation of ophthalmoscopic changes of hypertension and arteriolar sclerosis. *Arch Ophthalmol* **49:**117–138, 1953.

    A classic reference that discusses the grading of the retinopathy associated with hypertension and arteriolar sclerosis.

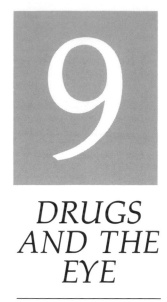

DRUGS
AND THE
EYE

Objectives

As a primary care physician, you should be able to use drugs to facilitate an eye examination, including how to stain the corneal surface with fluorescein, anesthetize the cornea with a topical anesthetic, and dilate the pupil with one or more mydriatic drugs. You should be aware of potential ocular complications of eye drops and systemic drugs you might prescribe, and recognize these ocular complications when they do occur. In addition, you should be able to interpret the systemic effects of the topical ophthalmic drugs that an ophthalmologist might prescribe for your patients.

To achieve these objectives you should learn:

- The technique of applying drugs to the conjunctival sac.
- The ocular effects and complications of topical ocular anesthetics, mydriatics, and corticosteroids. *(See cautions regarding dilating the pupil in Chapter 1, The Eye Examination, and the therapeutic warnings regarding topical anesthetics and topical corticosteroids in Chapter 4, Red Eye.)*
- The ocular side effects of systemically administered corticosteroids, the chloroquines, digitalis, diphenylhydantoin, ethambutol, and the phenothiazines.
- The systemic side effects of the beta-adrenergic blockers, the cholinergic-stimulators, and the adrenergic drugs.

Relevance

You will need to use diagnostic drugs in order to perform a complete ocular examination, skills that every primary care physician should possess. You must be familiar with the side effects and complications of diagnostic and therapeutic drugs in order to avoid them when possible and to recognize them when they do occur.

Basic Information

Diagnostic Drugs

The following are drugs used to execute a complete eye examination.

Fluorescein. Sodium fluorescein *(Ful-Glo®)* is a water soluble dye that produces an orange-yellow fluorescent color when applied to the conjunctival sac. When viewed under cobalt blue or fluorescent light, the color is a brilliant green. It is not irritating to the eye and is extremely helpful in detecting abrasions of the corneal surface since fluorescein stains damaged epithelium *(see Chapter 1, The Eye Examination, Fig. 5).* A sterile, individually packaged dry fluorescein strip is moistened with a drop of sterile water or saline and then applied to the inferior bulbar conjunctiva. A few blinks spread the now visible tear film across the cornea. Although there are no systemic complications that attend the use of topical fluorescein, the porous structure of a soft contact lens will absorb the dye. To avoid discoloration, contact lenses should be removed before the fluorescein is applied.

Topical anesthetics. Among the topical anesthetics, the most widely used is proparacaine hydrochloride 0.5% *(Ak-taine®, Alcaine®, Ophthaine®, Ophthetic®).* The instillation of one drop of this surface-active compound renders the corneal epithelium insensate within fifteen seconds. Such anesthesia is useful to make surface manipulations painless, for example, removing a superficial corneal foreign body or performing Schiotz tonometry. It also facilitates the examination of a damaged painful cornea that otherwise might be difficult because of the pain. Topical anesthetics rarely produce local or systemic allergy. They should never be prescribed for repeated use by patients because they are toxic to the corneal epithelium; they inhibit mitosis and cellular migration, and can lead to corneal ulceration and permanent corneal scarring.

Mydriatics. Mydriatics are drugs that dilate the pupil. There are only two classes of mydriatics.

- *Cholinergic-blocking (or parasympatholytic) drugs.* Drugs in this category dilate the pupil by paralyzing the iris sphincter. There are several such drugs in regular use: tropicamide 1% *(Mydriacyl®, Tropicacyl®);* cyclopentolate hydrochloride 1% *(AK-pentolate®, Cyclogyl®);* and homatropine hydrobromide 2% *(Homatrocel®, Isopto® Homatropine).* Atropine sulfate 1% *(Atropisol®)* and scopolamine hydrobromide 0.25% *(Isopto® Hyoscine)* are also available for topical ocular use, but they should never be used just to dilate the pupil, because they may last one to two weeks.

This class of drugs produces not only mydriasis, but cycloplegia, or paralysis of the muscles of the ciliary body. For this reason, these drugs are often referred to as cycloplegics. Cycloplegia produces paralysis of accommodation; therefore, the patient's reading vision may be blurred until these drugs wear off. Nevertheless, these drugs are widely employed by physicians because they produce excellent mydriasis. Tropicamide is the most popular mydriatic with primary care physicians and ophthalmologists alike because of its rapid onset and short duration. It produces its maximum pupillary dilation thirty minutes after instillation, and the effect is spent within four to five hours. Cautions regarding pupillary dilation are discussed in *Chapter 1, The Eye Examination.* Systemic side effects of tropicamide are decidedly rare because of its brief duration of action, but they may be serious. They include nausea, vomiting, pallor, and vasomotor collapse.

- *Adrenergic-stimulating (or sympathomimetic) drugs.* These drugs dilate the pupil by stimulating the pupillary dilator muscle. There is only one such drug in regular use: phenylephrine hydrochloride 2.5% *(Efricel®, Neo-Synephrine®).* One drop applied to the eye dilates the pupil in thirty to forty minutes, but has no effect on accommodation (hence the statement that phenylephrine is a mydriatic, but not a cycloplegic drug). This means that the patient can still read after the use of this drug. However, the mydriasis produced is neither as rapid nor as great as with tropicamide, and the pupil remains reactive to light. For these reasons, phenylephrine is seldom used alone as a mydriatic.

When maximum mydriasis is required, for example, when the far periphery of the retina must be examined, phenylephrine in combination with tropicamide is ideal because the effects are additive. This combination is often used to dilate the pupil of a brown iris as well, because mydriatics are less effective in dark-eyed individuals as compared to blue-eyed ones. The 2.5% solution of phenylephrine is much preferred to the 10% solution, because the stronger preparation has been associated with acute hypertension and even with myocardial infarction in some patients. In infants, the combination of cyclopentolate hydrochloride 0.2% and phenylephrine hydrochloride 1.0% *(Cyclomydril®)* is safe and effective.

Topical Ocular Drugs

The following are topically applied ocular drugs of clinical importance.

Ocular decongestants. This group of drugs is important if only because more than a million bottles of ocular decongestant are purchased each month in the United States. These are topically applied, weak adrenergic-stimulating drugs, which temporarily whiten the eye through their vasoconstrictor effect. They are advertised as effective in relieving redness of the eye due to minor eye irritations caused by smoke, dust, smog, wind, glare, swimming, and contact lenses.

The over-the-counter brands of these drugs will be familiar to most readers. Naphazoline hydrochloride 0.012% *(Degest II®, Clear Eyes®),* phenylephrine hydrochloride 0.12% *(Eye Cool®, Velva Kleen®),* and tetrahydrozaline hydrochloride 0.05% *(Murine® Plus, Visine®)* are the three major drugs in this category. There is a widespread belief among laymen that the use of these compounds is part of good ocular hygiene. This is a misconception. Red, tired, burning eyes will likely benefit as much from a cold, wet compress to the closed eyelids as they would from these compounds. Nevertheless, these compounds are sold in high volume.

The most frequent complication of their use arises from their overuse: rebound vasodilation of conjunctival vessels. In other words, when used to excess, ocular decongestants can cause an increase rather than a decrease in redness of the eyes. In rare instances, acute angle-closure glaucoma may be precipitated by the use of sympathomimetic drugs in susceptible eyes, because they can dilate the pupil. However, they may be used without harm by patients with chronic open-angle glaucoma, because they do not produce a rise in pressure if the filtration angle is open.

Topical ocular corticosteroids. Topical corticosteroids never should be prescribed by a primary care physician unless there is a precise indication for their use, for example, acute or chronic iritis. The serious complications of this class of drugs are discussed in *Chapter 1, Red Eye.* To reiterate, topical corticosteroids may promote infections by viruses, bacteria, and fungi. They also lead to the development of glaucoma and cataracts. Avoid using topical corticosteroids unless you have an exact ocular diagnosis for which they are indicated.

Ocular Side Effects

The drugs discussed below are systemically administered medications that may have profound ocular or neuro-ocular effects.

Corticosteroids. Corticosteroids, or more properly, adrenocorticosteroids, when given long term in moderate dosage, produce posterior subcapsular cataracts. Asthmatic children, post–renal-transplant patients, and adults with rheumatoid arthritis are groups in which this phenomenon has been commonly observed. Patients with rheumatoid arthritis may develop posterior subcapsular cataracts in the absence of corticosteroid therapy, but the incidence increases with corticosteroid therapy.

The chloroquines. Chloroquine phosphate *(Aralen®)* and hydroxychloroquine sulfate *(Plaquenil®)*, originally used in the treatment of malaria, are now also used to treat rheumatoid arthritis, lupus erythematosus, and some rare dermatologic disorders. Chloroquines can produce corneal deposits and retinopathy. The corneal deposits are usually asymptomatic, but can produce glare and photophobia (ocular discomfort in bright lights); the deposits regress when the drug is discontinued. The retinopathy is much more serious. This drug-induced retinal damage is insidious, slowly progressive, and usually irreversible. The typical bull's eye macular lesions do not become visible ophthalmoscopically until serious retinal damage has already occurred. Patients on high dosages of drugs (for example, more than 250 mg a day of chloroquine phosphate) or on long-term treatment (for example, three or more years with at least 300 grams total dose of chloroquine phosphate) are at the greatest risk. Patients using the chloroquines require regular ophthalmological examinations, with visual acuity, color vision, visual field, and ophthalmoscopic testing at the minimum.

Digitalis. Intoxication with this widely used cardiovascular drug almost always produces blurred and/or abnormally colored vision (i.e., chromatopsia). Classically, normal objects appear yellow with the overdosage of digitalis, but green, red, brown, or blue vision can also occur. White halos may be perceived on dark objects, or objects may seem frosted in appearance. Usually, there is a concomitant development of fatigue and weakness with digitalis intoxication, but the visual disturbances often dominate the patient's complaints.

Diphenylhydantoin. Still widely used for the control of seizures, diphenylhydantoin sodium *(Dilantin®)* causes dose-related cerebellar-vestibular effects. Horizontal nystagmus in lateral gaze with vertical nystagmus in up gaze, vertigo, ataxia, and even diplopia will occur with mildly elevated blood levels. More complex forms of nystagmus and even ophthalmoplegia may complicate extremely elevated blood levels. These effects are reversible when the intoxication is reversed.

Ethambutol. Ethambutol is a drug useful in the chemotherapy of tuberculosis. As a side effect, ethambutol produces a dose-related optic neuropathy. With dosages of 15 mg/kg/day, optic neuropathy occurs in less than one percent of patients, but increases to five percent of patients receiving 25 mg/kg/day and to fifteen percent receiving 50 mg/kg/day. The onset of visual loss may be within one month of starting the drug. Recovery usually occurs when the drug is stopped, but it may take months; occasionally, visual loss is permanent.

Phenothiazines

- *Chlorpromazine.* This psychoactive drug produces punctate opacities in the corneal epithelium after long-term dosage. Occasionally, opacities develop on the lens surface as well. These opacities are reversible with discontinuation of the drug.

- *Thioridazine.* Thioridazine, commonly used to treat patients with psychosis, produces a pigmentary retinopathy after high dosage, usually at least 1000 mg/day. Hence, the current recommendation of 800 mg/day as the maximum dose.

Systemic Side Effects

The drugs discussed below are topically administered ocular drugs. These drugs usually are employed in the treatment of glaucoma, and all have rather potent systemic side effects.

Beta-Adrenergic Blockers

Timolol and levobunolol. Nonselective beta-adrenergic antagonists, timolol maleate *(Timoptic®)* and levobunolol hydrochloride *(Betagan®)* reduce the formation of aqueous humor by the ciliary body and thereby reduce intraocular pressure. Timolol and its analog levobunolol are very effective and widely used. Side effects include bronchospasm. Thus, these drugs are contraindicated in patients with asthma or chronic obstructive pulmonary disease. Several deaths have been reported secondary to the pulmonary complications of topically administered timolol. Because of their cardiac effects, topical timolol or levobunolol may precipitate or worsen cardiac failure, and must be used with caution if bradycardia or systemic hypotension will adversely affect the patient.

Betaxolol. A cardioselective beta-1-adrenergic antagonist, betaxolol hydrochloride *(Betoptic®)* was developed to avoid the pulmonary complications of timolol. Introduced in 1985, betaxolol may be as effective as timolol in lowering intraocular pressure without the pulmonary side effects. However, pulmonary effects have occasionally been noted, and caution should be used when this drug is employed in patients with excessive restriction of pulmonary function.

Cholinergic-Stimulating Drugs

Pilocarpine. Pilocarpine hydrochloride *(Isopto® Carpine)* is still widely used in the treatment of glaucoma. The systemic toxicity of pilocarpine is rare because it takes five to ten times the usual dose used for the treatment of open-angle glaucoma (i.e., one drop in each eye) to produce systemic effects. Nevertheless, toxicity occurs occasionally. Lacrimation, salivation, perspiration, nausea, vomiting, and diarrhea are seen with pilocarpine overdosage.

Echothiophate. A long-acting anticholinesterase, echothiophate iodide *(Phospholine Iodide®)* also mimics stimulation of the parasympathetic nervous system and is, therefore, in clinical use in the treatment of glaucoma, and also occasionally in the treatment of accommodative esotropia. Its side effects are identical to those described for pilocarpine. In addition, since chronic use of this drug inactivates plasma cholinesterase, patients being treated with echothiophate are more susceptible to the toxic effects of succinylcholine and procaine, because plasma cholinesterase hydrolyzes those agents. Prolonged apnea and even death have been reported from the use of succinylcholine during anesthesia in a patient with a low blood cholinesterase secondary to treatment with topical ocular echothiophate.

Adrenergic Drugs

Epinephrine. Epinephrine hydrochloride *(Epifrin®, Glaucon®)* is still rather widely used in the treatment of glaucoma. In unusually sensitive patients, or when large amounts of epinephrine are systemically absorbed, the adrenergic stimulation can produce cardiac arrhythmias or an increase in systemic blood pressure.

Points to Remember

- *Point 1.* When administering eye drops, try not to think of the pupil as the "bull's eye" at which you must aim the drop. The center of the cornea is the single most sensitive part of the eye. Eyedrops should not be dropped directly on the central cornea. Instead, roll the lower lid down and release the drop into the lower conjunctival fornix, the least sensitive part of the surface of the eye.

- *Point 2.* Never use atropine or scopolamine to dilate the pupil for a fundus examination.
- *Point 3.* Never give a patient a prescription for a topical anesthetic (or a sample, either).
- *Point 4.* Never use or prescribe a topical ocular corticosteroid unless you have a precise diagnosis for which it is specifically indicated. You must be prepared to monitor the patient for the serious side effects, for example, glaucoma or cataract.

Sample Problems

1. A busy medical student comes to you in the midst of exam week because he is experiencing severe headaches. As part of a complete physical, you perform a basic eye examination. During ophthalmoscopy, you find that you cannot fully see the optic disc because of the patient's very small pupil size. You find no indications against dilating the pupil and decide to do so to facilitate ophthalmoscopy. Your patient is a brown-eyed male, twenty-five years of age and in excellent health. Which of the following drugs would you select to dilate the pupils?

   (a) phenylephrine hydrochloride 0.12%
   (b) phenylephrine hydrochloride 2.5%
   (c) phenylephrine hydrochloride 10%
   (d) atropine sulfate 1%
   (e) tropicamide + phenylephrine hydrochloride 2.5%

   Answer: Choice (b). The patient is experiencing severe headaches. A potential source of these headaches is increased intracranial pressure due to brain tumor, with resultant papilledema. Therefore, it is important to see the optic disc clearly to examine for these findings. Atropine sulfate 1% is never used for simple pupillary dilation because its effects may last one to two weeks. The 0.12% solution of phenylephrine is the strength found in many over-the-counter ocular decongestants. The 10% solution is not the preferred concentration since it may be associated with serious systemic side effects in certain individuals. Occasionally, phenylephrine 2.5% will not provide sufficient dilation in brown-eyed individuals, and tropicamide and phenylephrine must be used. However, the physician can make this decision as he proceeds with the examination, particularly in situations where the patient would prefer to have the dilation subside quickly to allow clear vision.

2. A patient who has recently moved to the area is referred to you by a friend. He comes to you because he's been feeling especially tired lately and is easily fatigued after only minor activity. He is also concerned about his vision; things seem "dingy or yellow" to him lately. He's not exactly sure when this started. He has a history of heart disease and takes cardiac medications. Examination reveals no health problems, other than his heart condition, which appears stable. He asks if you think he should see an ophthalmologist about his eyes. What do you tell him?

Answer: Symptoms of blurred and/or abnormally colored vision occur with digitalis intoxication. Yellow vision is classic, but green, red, brown, or blue vision also can occur. Some patients perceive white halos on dark objects, or objects may look frosted. Fatigue and weakness are also characteristic. Usually such symptoms only occur with overdosage and stop with discontinuation of the drug. Since no other health problems exist, it is safe to assume that his symptoms are due to digitalis intoxication and are temporary. The step to take in this case is to reduce the dose of digitalis given to the patient until the visual symptoms and fatigue are eliminated. The patient should be monitored during the recovery period, but referral to an ophthalmologist is not necessary since the visual symptoms have been explained.

Annotated References

1. Ellis PP: *Ocular Therapeutics and Pharmacology,* ed 6. St. Louis, Mo, CV Mosby Co, 1981.

   A small book written by an author with a wealth of experience in ocular pharmacology and complications.

2. Fraunfelder FT, Roy FH: *Current Ocular Therapy 2.* Philadelphia, WB Saunders Co, 1985.

   An extensive text written by approximately seventy contributing authors and edited by two experienced ophthalmologists. Coverage is very wide and fairly detailed, with a good emphasis on drug complications.

3. Gilman AG, Goodman LS, Rall TW, et al (eds): *Goodman and Gilman's The Pharmacologic Basis of Therapeutics,* ed 7. New York, Macmillan, 1985.

   One of the best basic science text books on drugs. Serves as an encyclopedic reference on drugs in general.

4. Grant WM: *Toxicology of the Eye,* ed 3. Springfield, Ill, CC Thomas, 1986.

   Another encyclopedic treatment. A prodigious and scholarly work, carefully documenting ocular and neuro-ocular side effects of enumerable chemicals and drugs.

5. Havener WH: *Ocular Pharmacology,* ed 5. St. Louis, CV Mosby Co, 1983.

   An amiable and user-friendly book by an experienced ophthalmologist/ retinal surgeon with an abiding interest in basic pharmacology. Good emphasis on side effects and complications.

6. *Physicians' Desk Reference for Ophthalmology,* ed 14. Oradell, NJ, Medical Economics Co, 1986.

   A slim volume distilling from the parent PDR those drugs used by ophthalmologists. Like the parent volume, the package insert for each drug is reproduced for each of the pharmaceuticals. In addition, there are supplementary charts, tables, and flow sheets of use to clinicians. There is a section on ophthalmic lenses, one on visual standards and low vision, and a reprinting of the American Medical Association's Guide to the Evaluation of Permanent Visual Impairment. There is also an appendix with a glossary of ophthalmic terms and abbreviations.

INDEX

Numbers in bold face refer to pages that contain either a table, photo, illustration, or figure, alone or accompanied by text.

B

Diphenylhydantoin, 144
Diplopia, 79, 83, **87**, 99, 109, 111, 114–115, 116, 122, 123, 134, 144
Discharge, **62**, 63, 67, **68**, 71, 74, 75, see also Exudation
Dot hemorrhage, 126, **128**, **129**
Double vision, see Diplopia
Drugs, and the eye, see Ocular drugs
Drusen, **50**, **51**, 53, 55, 56
Dry eyes, 60, 67

E

Echothiophate, 145
Edema
  conjunctival, **65**
  corneal, 27, 60, 63, **64**, 66, 70, 76, **85**
  eyelid, 134
  macular, 126, 127
  optic disc, 43, 118
  optic nerve, 131
  retinal, 133
Epicanthus, **105**, 108
Epinephrine, 145
Epiphora, 79
Episclera, 59
Episcleritis, 59, **61**
Erythema multiforme, 70
Esophoria, **99**
Esotropia, **99**, **100**, **104**, **105**, 106, 108, 145
Ethambutol, 144
Exophoria, **99**
Exophthalmos, 133, **134**
Exotropia, **99**, **100**
Extraocular muscles, 2, **2B**
Exudates, 126, 127, **128**, 130, 131, 132, 133, 138
Exudation, **69**, 70, see also Discharge
Eye
  anatomy of, **2–3**, 79–81
  and central nervous system, 110
  cross-section of, **2A**
  drugs and, 140–147, see also Ocular drugs
  external landmarks, **2B**
  function of, 79–81
  injuries to, 78–94
  medications, 90, see also Ocular drugs
  misalignment of, see Strabismus; see also Diplopia
  ocular motility, see Eye movement
  ocular structures, **2–3**
  pigment, 15, **16**, 18

155

H

I

JKL

M

Mydriatics, **5**, 140, 141–142
Myelination, **17**, 18
Myopia, 15, 23, 47, 127, 130

161

ischemic damage to, 119
  lesion in, 26, 122, 123–124
  temporal pallor of, 42, **44**
  trauma to, 35
Optic neuritis, 32–33, 118, 119, 123
Optic neuropathy, 144
Optics, 3–4
Optometrist, xi
Orbit, 79, 82, **83**
Orbital hematoma, 83

P

Pain, **69**, 70, 80, 82, 88, 93
Palpation, 41, 42, 82, 92
Panretinal argon laser photocoagulation **129**
Papilledema, **17**, 33, **34**, 43, 117, 118, 119, 133, 146
Papillitis, **33**, 34, 118
Paralytic strabismus, 97, **98**
Parasympatholytic drugs, 141–142
Parinaud's oculoglandular syndrome, 67
Patching, **90**–91, 93, 97, 106, 109
Penlight, **5**
Penlight examination, 7, 26, 76, 77, 82, 84, 103, 108, **113**, 123
Perimetry, 43
Peripheral vision, 26, 34, 40
Perivasculitis, 135
Phenothiazines, 144
Photophobia, **69**, 70, 80, 143
Physiologic cup, 15, **16**, 41, 42, **43**, **44**
Picture card, **101**
Pigment crescent, 15, **16**
Pigment epithelial degeneration, 51, **52**
Pigment epithelial detachment, 81
Pilocarpine, 145
Pinhole, 6, 23, 24, 123
Posterior chamber, **2A**, 3, **40**
Preauricular adenopathy, 75
Preauricular lymph node, 67, **68**, 74
Preproliferative diabetic retinopathy, 126, **128**, **129**, 130
Presbyopia, 3–4, 9, 21
Proliferative diabetic retinopathy, 126–127, **129**, 130, 138
Proptosis, 63, **65**, 67, **68**, 83
Pseudoisochromatic plates, 10
Pseudopapilledema, 117, **118**
Pterygium, 59, **62**
Ptosis, **114**, **115**, 116, 122
Pulmonary complications of ocular drugs, 144–145

Retinal occlusion, **30**, 31, **32**, 35, 37
Retinal pigment epithelium, 15, 18, 50, 51, 53, 55
Retinal tears, 37, 92
Retinitis, 135, **136**
Retinoblastoma, **106**, 108
Retinopathy, 143, 144
  hypertensive, **132**
Retrobulbar optic neuritis, 33
Rheumatoid arthritis, 143
Rosenbaum pocket vision screener, **9**

S

Sarcoidosis, 125, 134–135
Scheie classification, **131**
Schiotz tonometer, **5**, 10, **12**, **13**, 14, 39, 63
  calibration scale for, **11**
Schiotz tonometry, 5, **12–13**, 14, 22, 26, 42, 44, 141
Schlemm's canal, **2A**, **40**, 41
Sclera, 2, **2A**, **2B**, 59, 81
Scleral crescent, **16**
Scleritis, 59, **61**
Scotoma, 29, 34, 40, 53, 55, 119, 121, 122
Seborrhea, 71, **72**
Seborrheic blepharitis, 71, **72**
Second sight, 47
Shield, **91**, 93
Single E chart, **101**
Snellen eye chart, 5, 6, **7**, 21, 63, 82, 102, 111, 127
Staphylococcal blepharitis, **71**
Steroids, 32, 33, 35
Stevens-Johnson syndrome, 70
Strabismus
  and amblyopia, 96, 97, 98
  classifications of, 97–99, **100**
  comitant, **97**, 98, 99, 102
  correcting, 106–107
  defined, 97
  early detection of, 107
  intermittent, 100, 108
  noncomitant, 97, **98**, 99, 102
  nonparalytic, **97**, 98
  paralytic, 97, **98**
  restrictive, 97, **98**
  surgery, 107, 134
  testing for, 100, 102, **103**, **104**, 105, 107, 108
Stye, 59, 72, **73**
Subconjunctival hemorrhage, 58, 59, 63, 72, 88, **89**

Subretinal hemorrhage, 51, **52**, 53
Subretinal neovascularization, 29, 50–51, **52**, 55, 126
Suturing, 91
Swinging flashlight test, 26, 111, 123, see also Penlight examination
Sympathetic ophthalmia, 91
Sympathomimetic drugs, 142, 143
Systemic disease, 2
    ocular manifestations of, 125–138

T

Tay-Sachs disease, 30
Tears, 79
Telangiectasias, 126, **128**
Temporal arteritis, 2, 34–35, 37, 123
Thioridazine, 144
Thyroid eye disease, 98, 125, 133–134
Thyroid stare, **134**
Timolol, 144
Tonometry, see Schiotz tonometry
Topical anesthetics, **5**, 12, 14, 74, 83, 88, 93, 140, 141, 146
Trabeculum, 41
Trauma, 27, 35, 36, **64**, 66, 77, 80, 81, 82, 83, 84, 91, 92, 115, 116, 135
Tuberculosis, 144
Tumor, 27, 106, 108, 124
    brain, 2, 42, 110, 115, 117, 118, 146

UVW

Upper respiratory infection, 70
Uveitis, 91, 135, 137
Vascular occlusions, 29–32, 37
Venous beading, **128**, **129**, 130
Viral conjunctivitis, 13, **68**, **69**, 70, 71, 72, 75
Vision
    defective, early treatment of, 102, 106, 107, see also Amblyopia
    development of, 96
Visual acuity
    and amblyopia, 95, 102, 107, 109
    and cataracts, 27, 45–48, 109, 127
    defined, 4
    and diabetes, 138
    and diabetic retinopathy, 126, 127, 130
    distance, 6
    estimating, in uncooperative patient, 10
    and glaucoma, 42

XYZ